MED

Medical engravings of the 19th century

PHILEMON STEIN

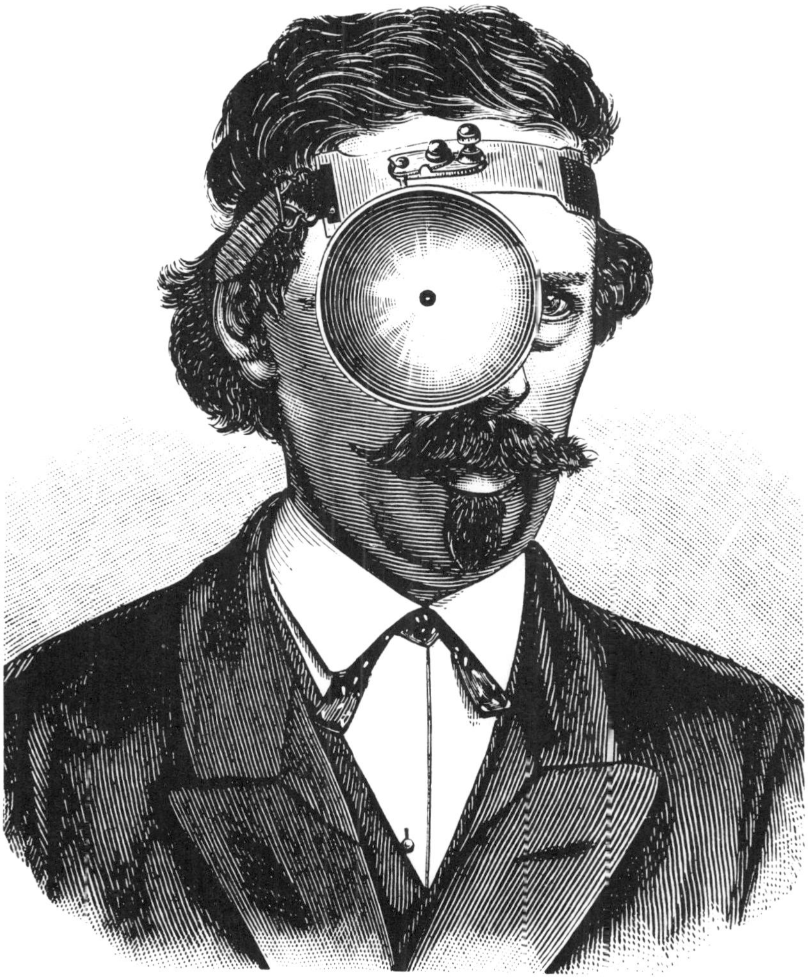

UNIVERSE BOOKS
New York

Published in the United States of America in 1974
by Universe Books
381 Park Avenue South, New York, N.Y. 10016

Library of Congress Card Number: 74-83562

Cloth edition: ISBN 0-87663-209-6
Paperback edition: ISBN 0-87663-914-7

Printed in the United States of America

This book is not intended solely for the medical corps.

The universal prevalence of illness illustrates the very essence of our being, since we all lie potentially in our sickbeds. It is therefore only justice that we be informed of certain exceptional cases rarely encountered by medicine in our time. And that is precisely what has been attempted here, by borrowing from medical publications of the XIXth century some of their best engravings.

In those days medicine was only concerned with preserving life, to the exclusion of all the esthetic factors that constitute such a large part of our happiness today. Congresses exhibited monstrosities to audiences of doctors in top hats. Nowadays the same monsters only appeal to side-show fanciers, whereas we unwittingly pass daily in the streets successfully corrected hare-lips and Siamese twins.

Medical art has become a science, essentially devoted to statistics, in other words to the majority. But the publications of these marginal cases gives rise to a sudden deep visual interest. The descriptive arts have also evolved, to the point where the absolute fidelity of color photography has removed all scientific value from the most beautiful of engravings. Graphic beauty is thus forever lost to science.

The engravings have been selected essentially according to esthetic values, and only secondarily for their fanciful appeal, excluding unhealthy voyeurism or disguised eroticism. External pathology is perceived directly by eyesight, since its only comparative bases are you and me. Therapy itself has undergone modifications pertaining more to form than to content. Dressed in white steel or chromium, miniaturized, it has followed the current laudable preoccupation with style. It always has. But what may be the reactions to our machines a century from now?

The absence of color, as well as the standardization of format, adds to the rigor required by such a work. There are few like it. It corresponds therefore to a real need, opening new horizons to the reader.

The engravings speak for themselves.

Dr. O. Blomquist

PARTIAL BIBLIOGRAPHY

Diccionario de Medicina. Madrid, 1880.
Haut und Geschlechtskrankheiten. Leipzig, 1894.
Der Lehrbuch der Chirurgie. Vienna, 1877.
Maladies du Testicule. Paris, 1857.
Das Neue Naturheitverfahren. Leipzig, 1897.
Voies Urinaires. Paris, 1855.

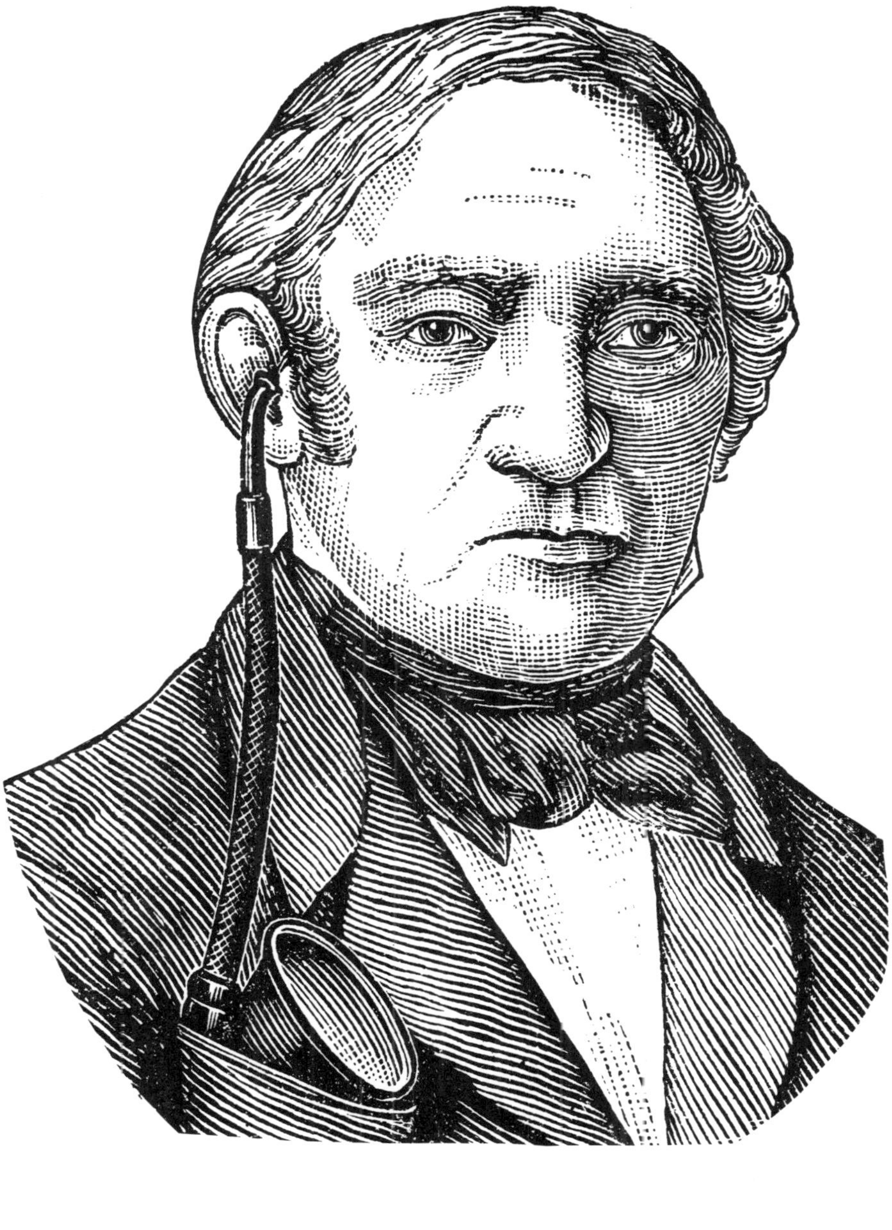

PATHOLOGIA

GYNECOLOGICAL EXAMINATION

Bezeman has ingeniously simplified speculum examinations. This distinguished practitioner has developed a speculum with which various operations on the uterus or the vaginal walls may be performed without any assistance whatsoever.

If, in the course of civilian practice, it becomes necessary to carry out a speculum examination in the patient's home, she should be placed across the bed and on its edge, so that her legs lie completely out of it. It is a good idea to place two or three folded sheets under her or, even better, a more solid body, a stool for instance, slipped between the mattresses, affording more resistance and keeping the pelvis from sinking into the bed. If two assistants are available, the examination is quite simple, as they can, by each holding one of the patient's feet, maintain her in the desired position. If no assistance is forthcoming, the doctor should sit in front of the patient and place her feet on each of his knees. If the prevalent conditions of daylight or artificial light are insufficient, an ordinary silver spoon behind a candle will do the trick.

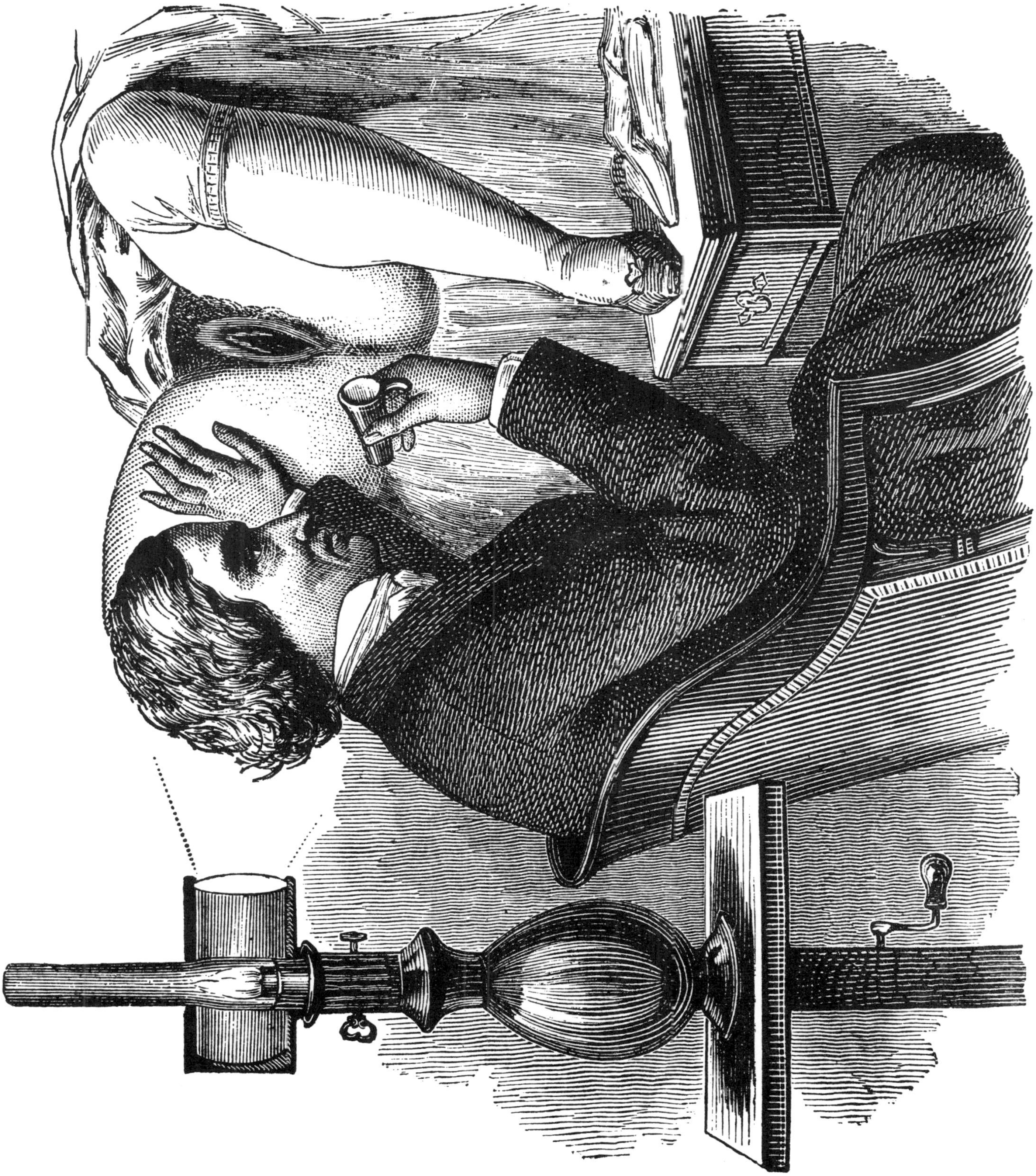

HYPERTROPHY OF THE BREAST

Bilateral hypertrophy of the breasts is an exceptional affliction. Cases in which breasts weighed more than forty pounds have been recorded.

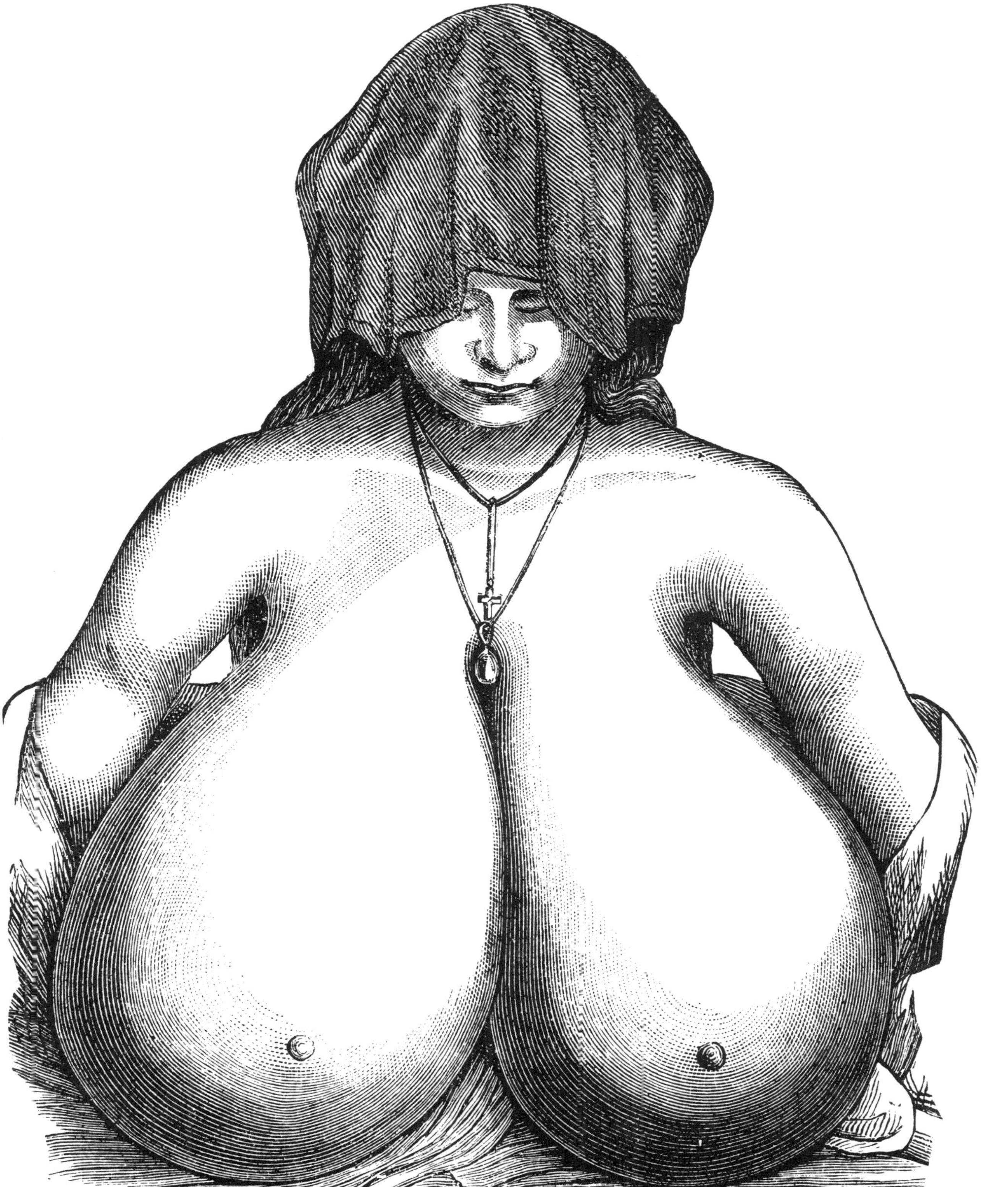

ELEPHANTIASIS OF THE SCROTUM

Elephantiasis of the scrotum produces a quite remarkable tumour. This ailment appears to be the result of a moderate skin inflammation, of a benign sort that, in hot climates, progressively brings about destructive modifications. The sickness begins with shivers followed by fever. The fever attacks are repeated at irregular intervals and after each one the swelling grows. The ordinarily healthy testicles are buried in the morbid mass, as is, finally, the penis. It is possible to live thus for years, in excellent health, with an enormous scrotum.

In St. Kitts, H. M. Wilkes removed a tumour from a Negro that weighed seventy nine kilograms, that was seventy five centimetres long, with a circumference of one metre eighty centimetres. Surgery lasted close to eight hours, each cut of the lancet yielding an abundant venous haemorrhage, and the patient died exhausted toward the end of the operation.

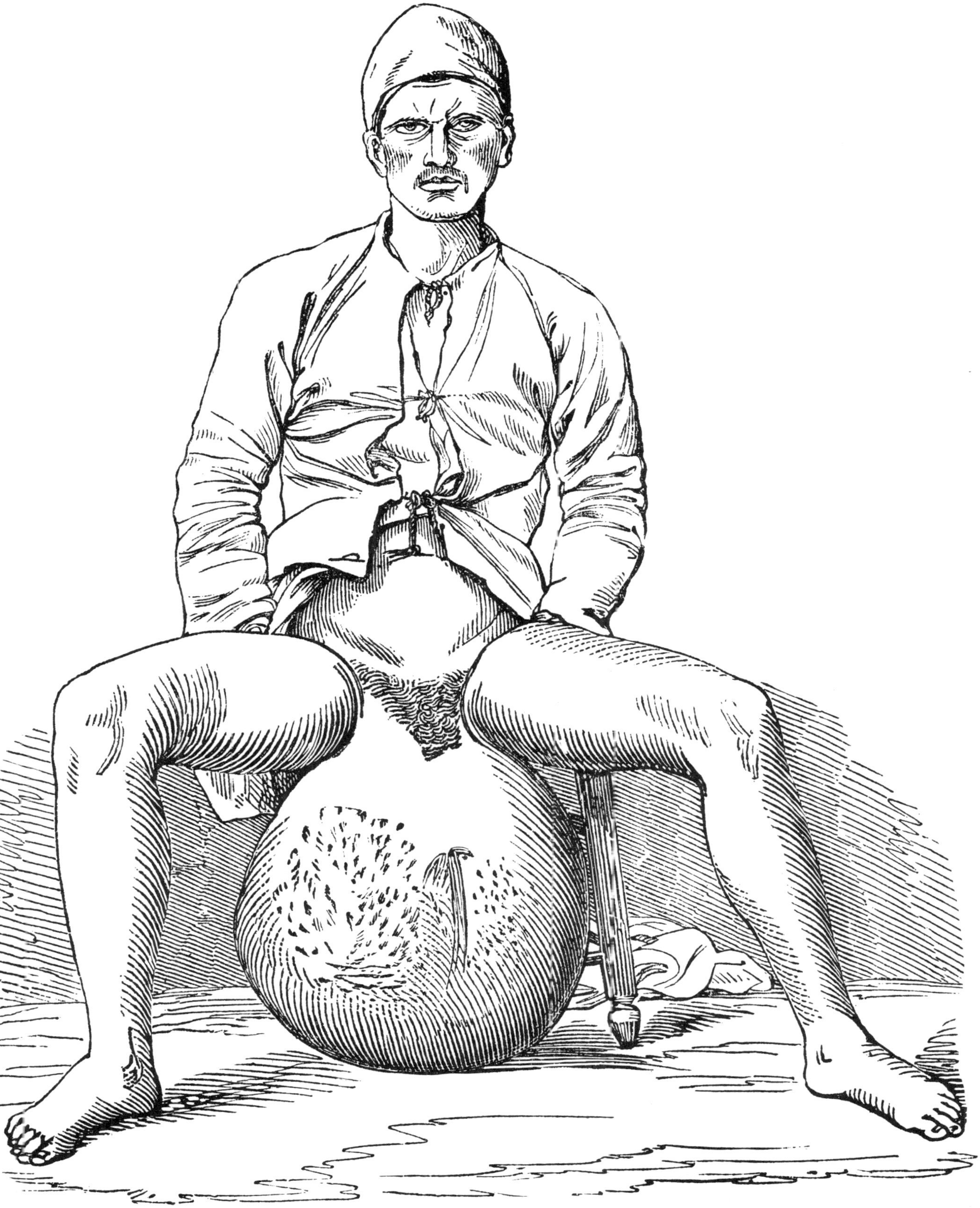

BREAST NAEVUS

The mark can vary in aspect from a small spot (birth-mark or mole) to a network of capillaries spread over a wide surface, or to a large cancerlike tumour.

This voluminous naevus, spread over a vast area of the front of the breast, resembles a malignant tumour. A small seton was introduced into this tumour, producing widespread gangrene which led to the obliteration of the veins.

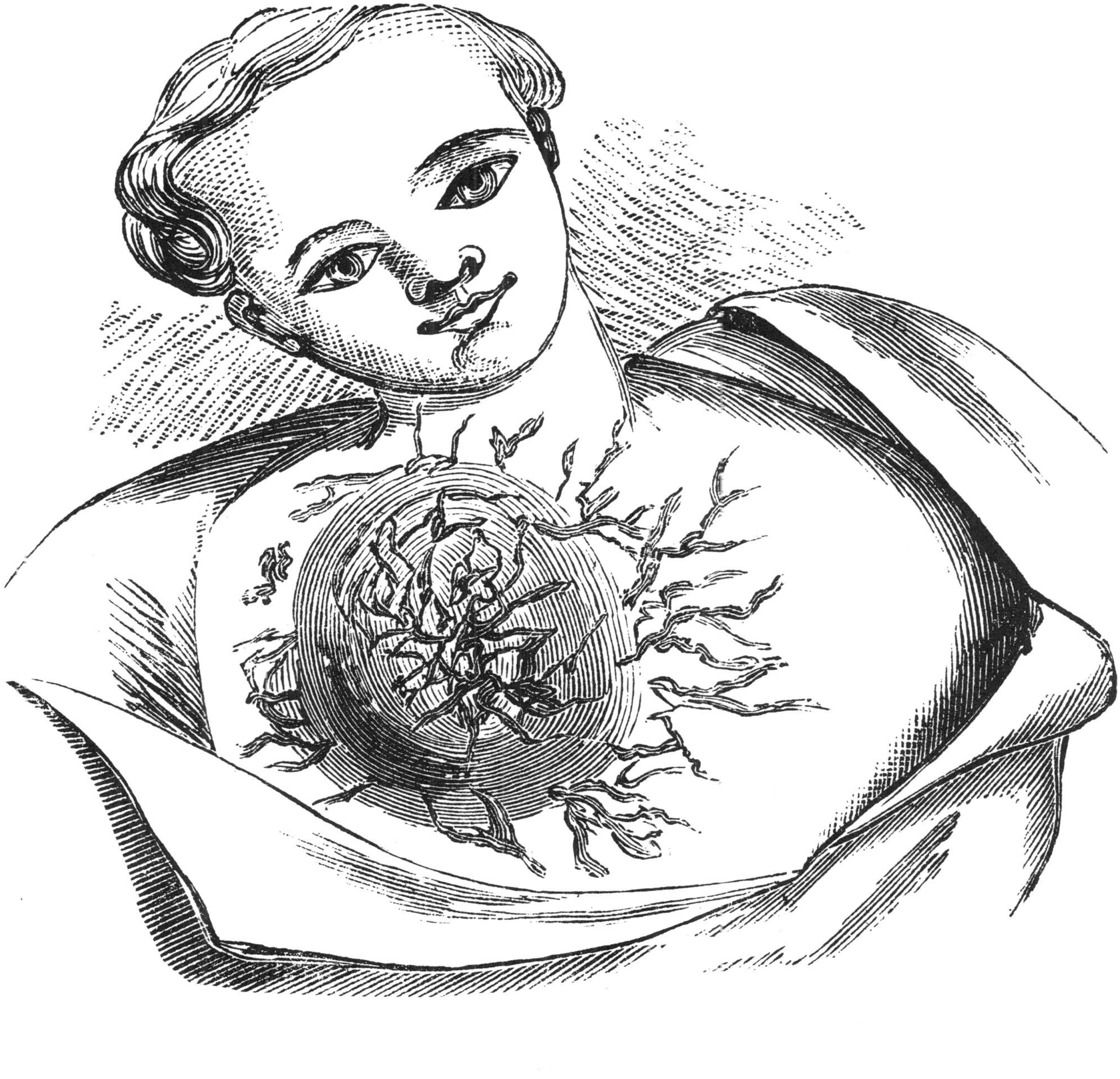

CYST OF THE OVARY

The cyst's development is slow and may take years. It usually appears between the ages of twenty and forty. Marriage and pregnancies seem to have no influence. Such a cyst can contain more than thirty litres of serum of gelatinous fluid. It can degenerate into a malignant, generalised, fatal tumour.

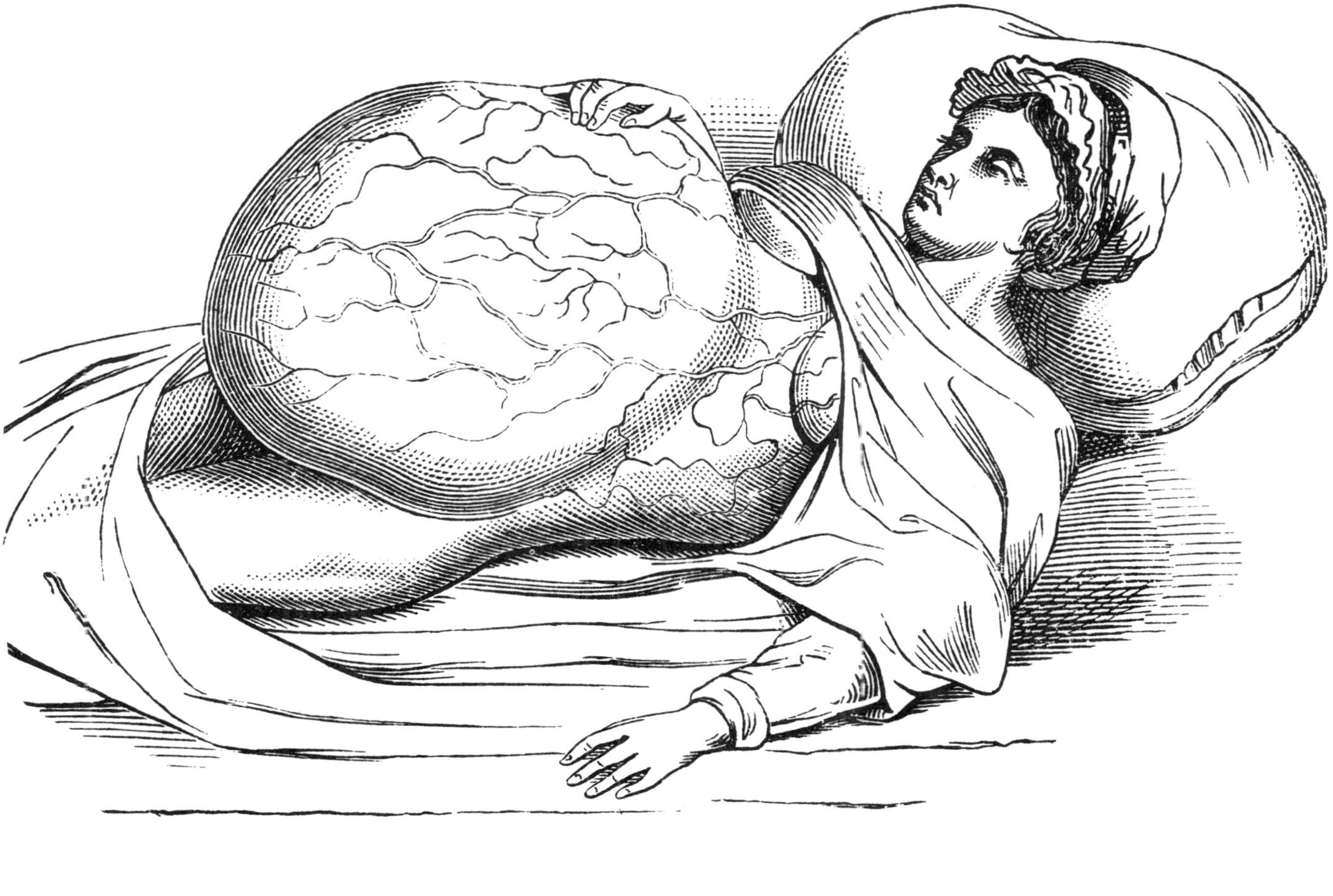

CHIRURGIA

COMPRESSIVE BANDAGING

A makeshift compressive bandage to stem a serious haemorrhage of the main artery of the left limb. The victim thus avoids losing all of his blood in the space of a few minutes.

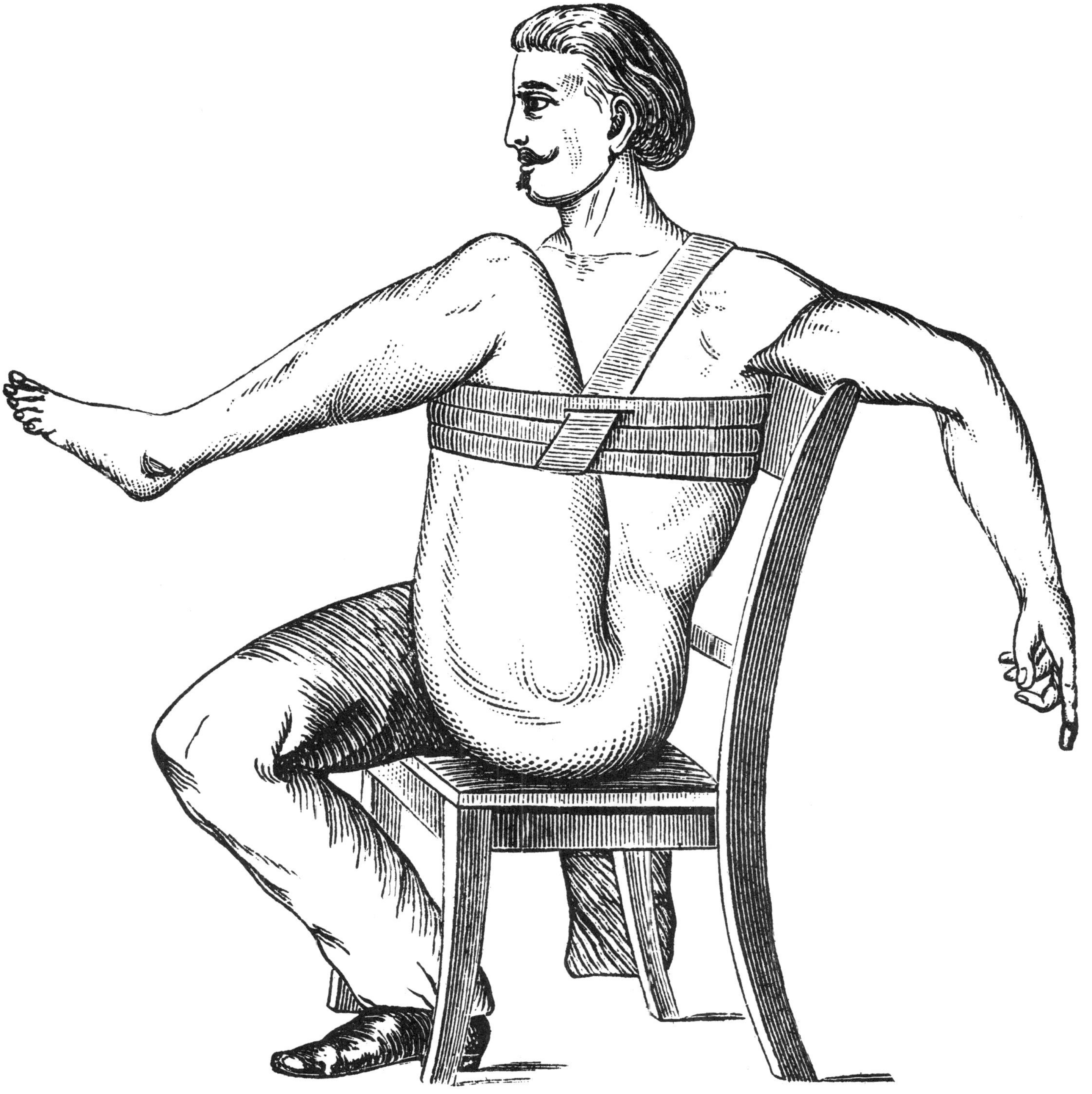

STRABISM OPERATION

The patient lying recumbent and chloroformed, the surgeon grasps a fold of the connective tissue on the interior rim of the cornea with the claw-forceps held in his left hand. He lifts the mucous membrane, incises with the point of the blunt scissors and, penetrating deeper, dissects the cellular tissue beneath. He then extricates with short little flips of the scissors the superior edge of the muscle under which he will soon want to slip the hook. The surgeon then introduces the large blunt hook, laid flat, through the opening in the connective tissue and twists it half-way around rotationally, with a certain amount of force; then, continuing to push energetically, he engages the curved part of the hook under the muscle, in an effort to enclose it completely. Once the hook is thus placed, he takes it in his left hand, pulling slightly so as to lift the tendon delicately up to the level of the insertion. He then detaches the tendon flush with the sclerotic.

During these manoeuvres, one should take care that the eyeball does not revolve, since in that case one might sever a tendon other than the one originally intended.

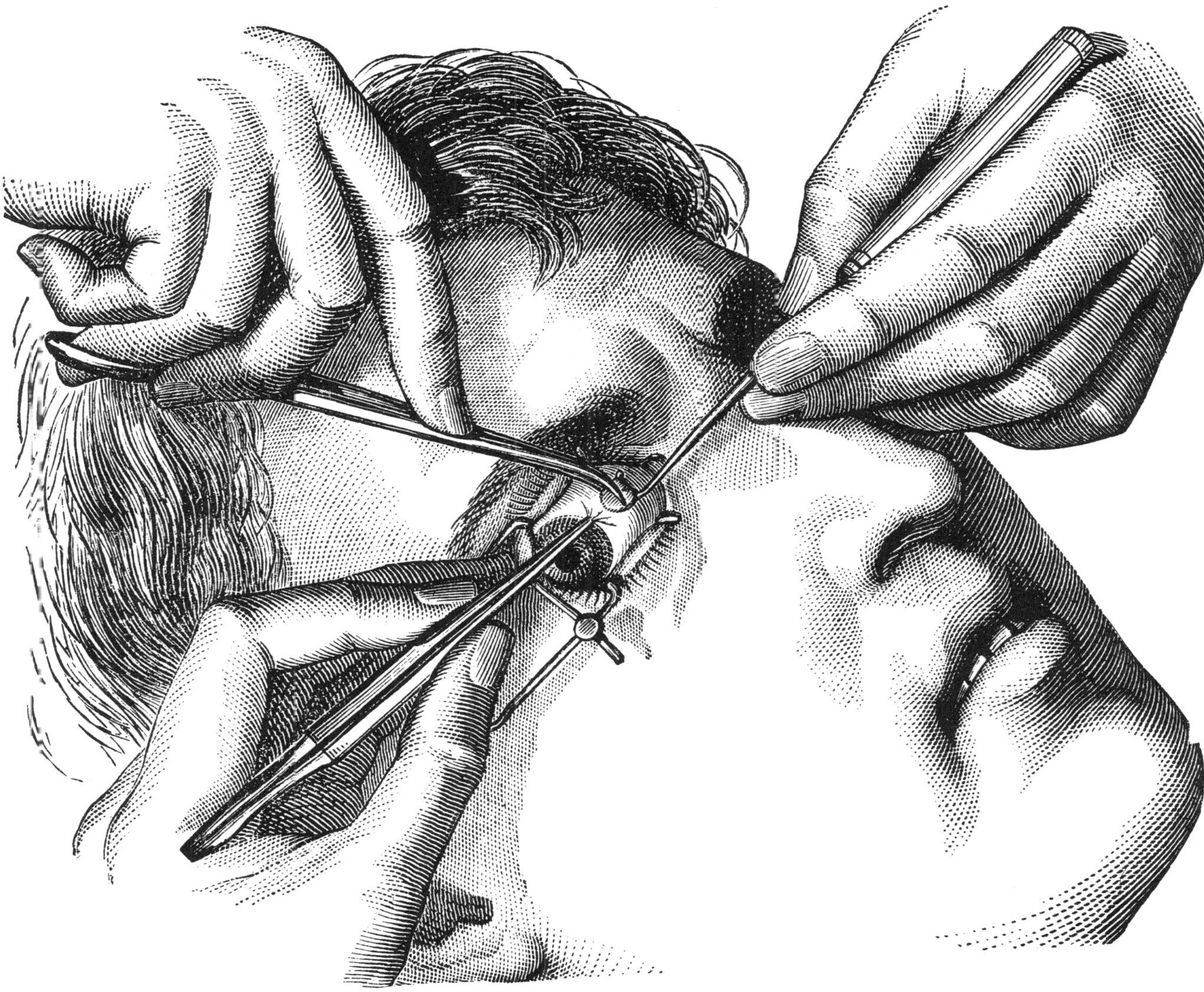

AUTOPSY

Removal of the sternum to facilitate access to the thoracic cavity and thus allow extraction and palpation of the lungs.

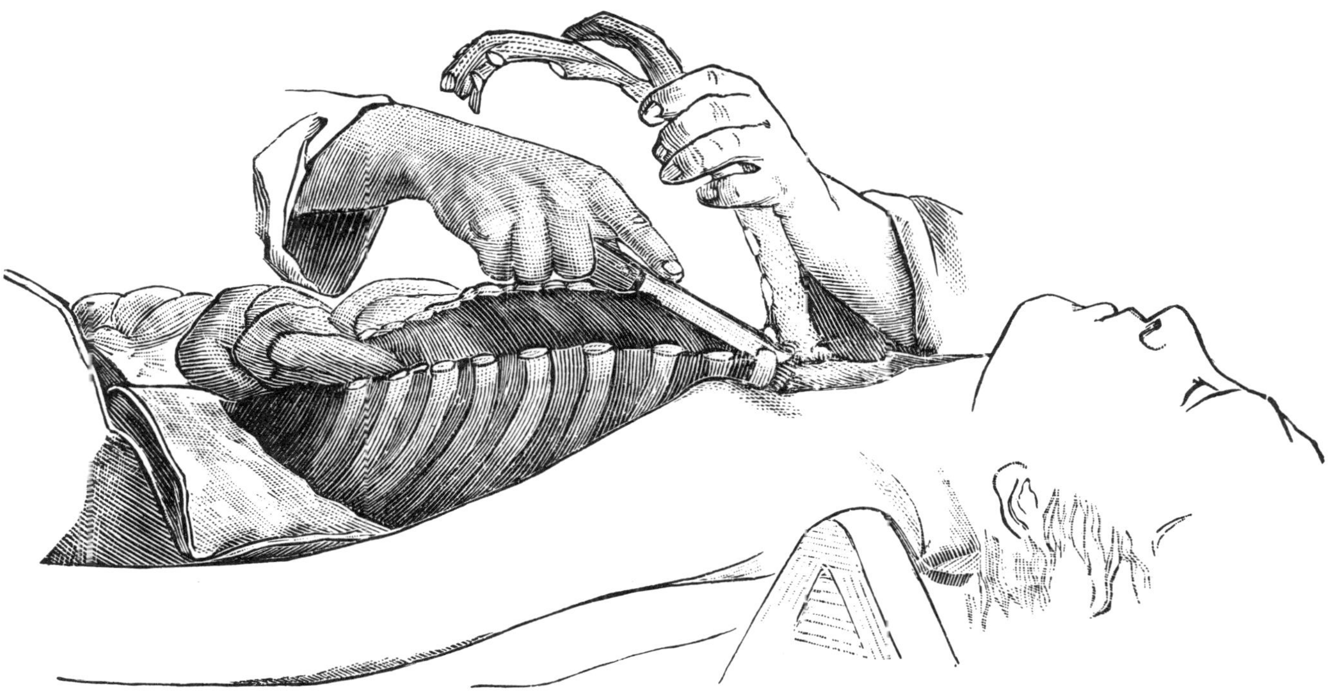

AMPUTATION OF THE LEG

Observe the various positions of the surgeon and his assistants. Before sawing through the bone, the surgeon sections the muscles.

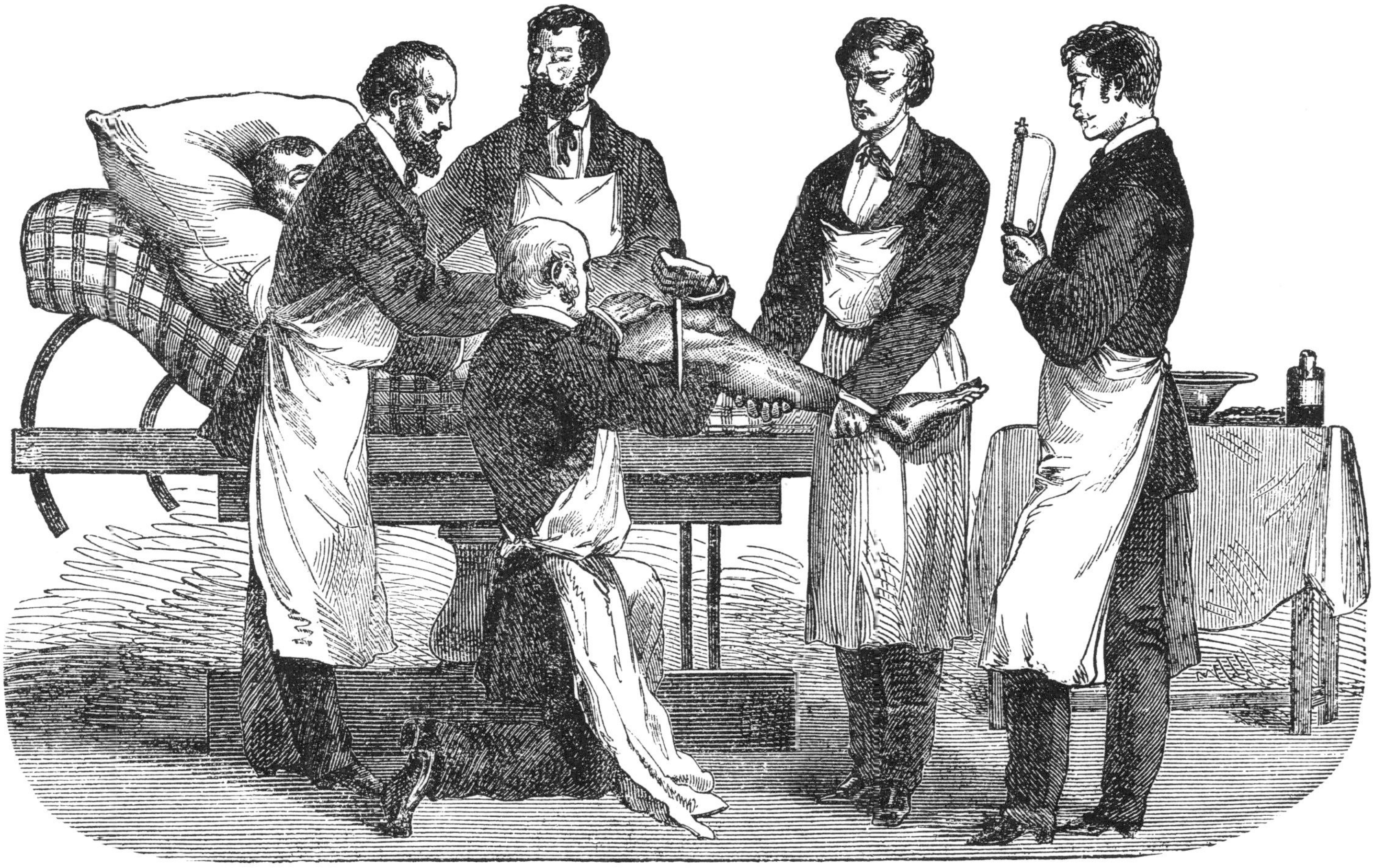

AMPUTATION OF THE THIGH

First stage of the amputation, incising the skin, a shred of which must be preserved in order to model the "stump".

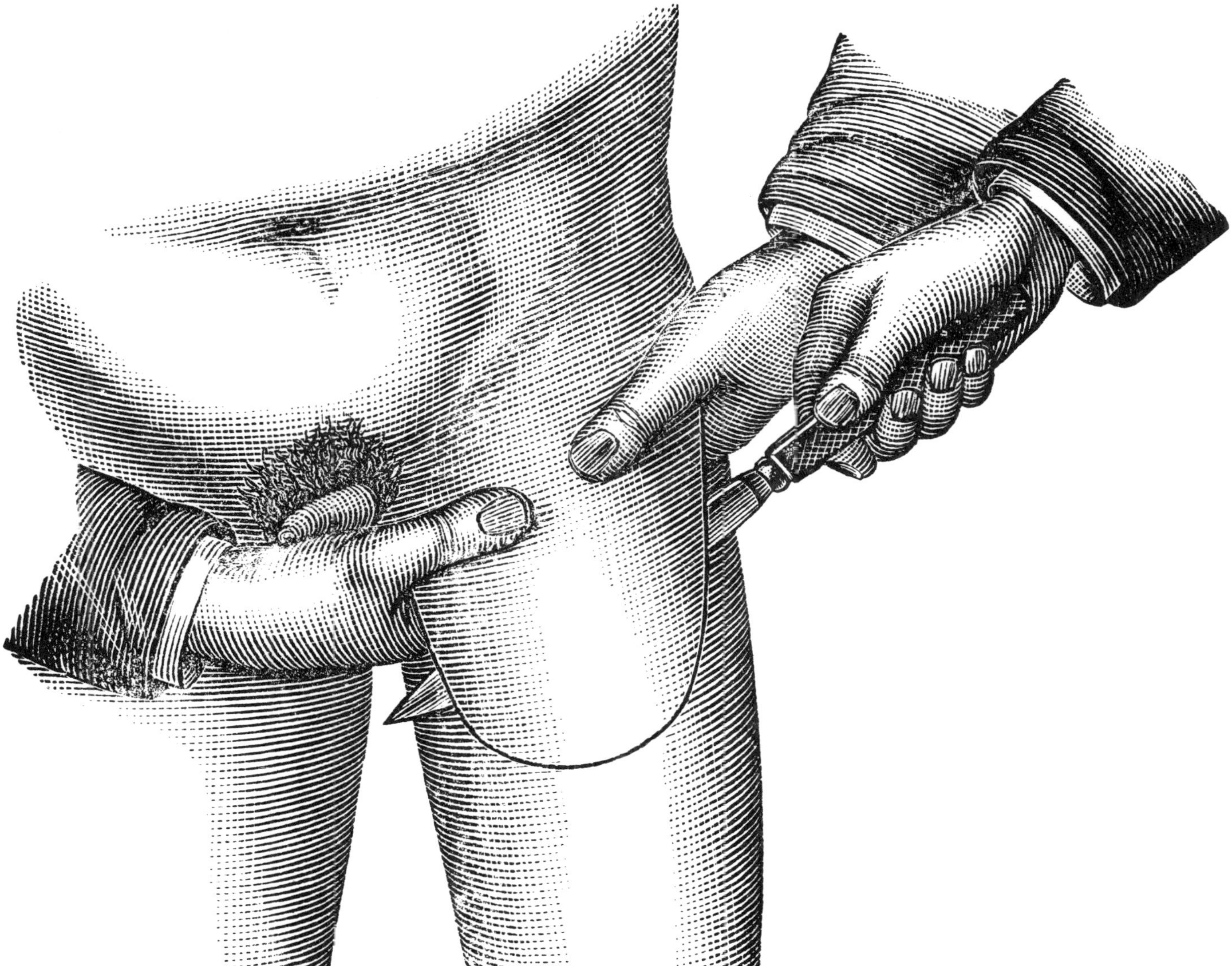

MODELLING THE STUMP

The operator holds the member to be sectioned firmly in one hand and, with the other, cuts the fleshy region under the articulation of the knee with a single stroke, grasping the knife firmly.

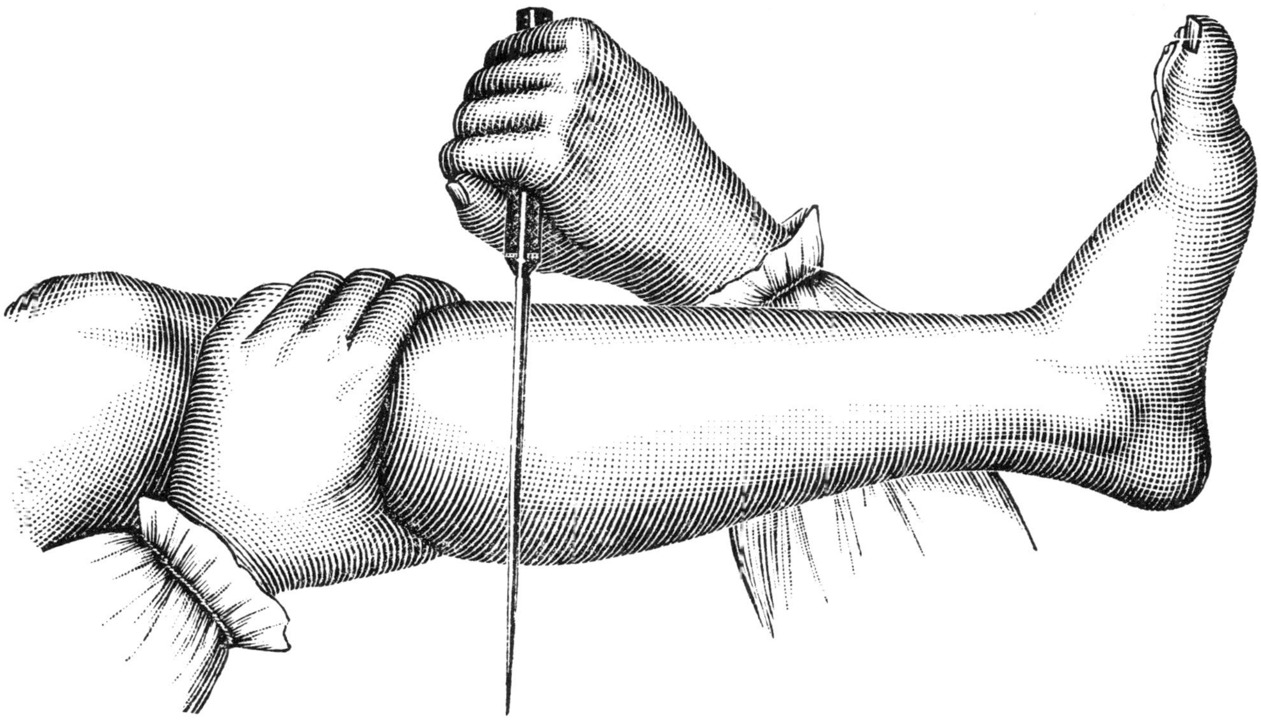

AMPUTATION OF THE FOOT

Firmly holding the inferior part of the foot in his left hand, the surgeon saws through the bone perpendicularly.

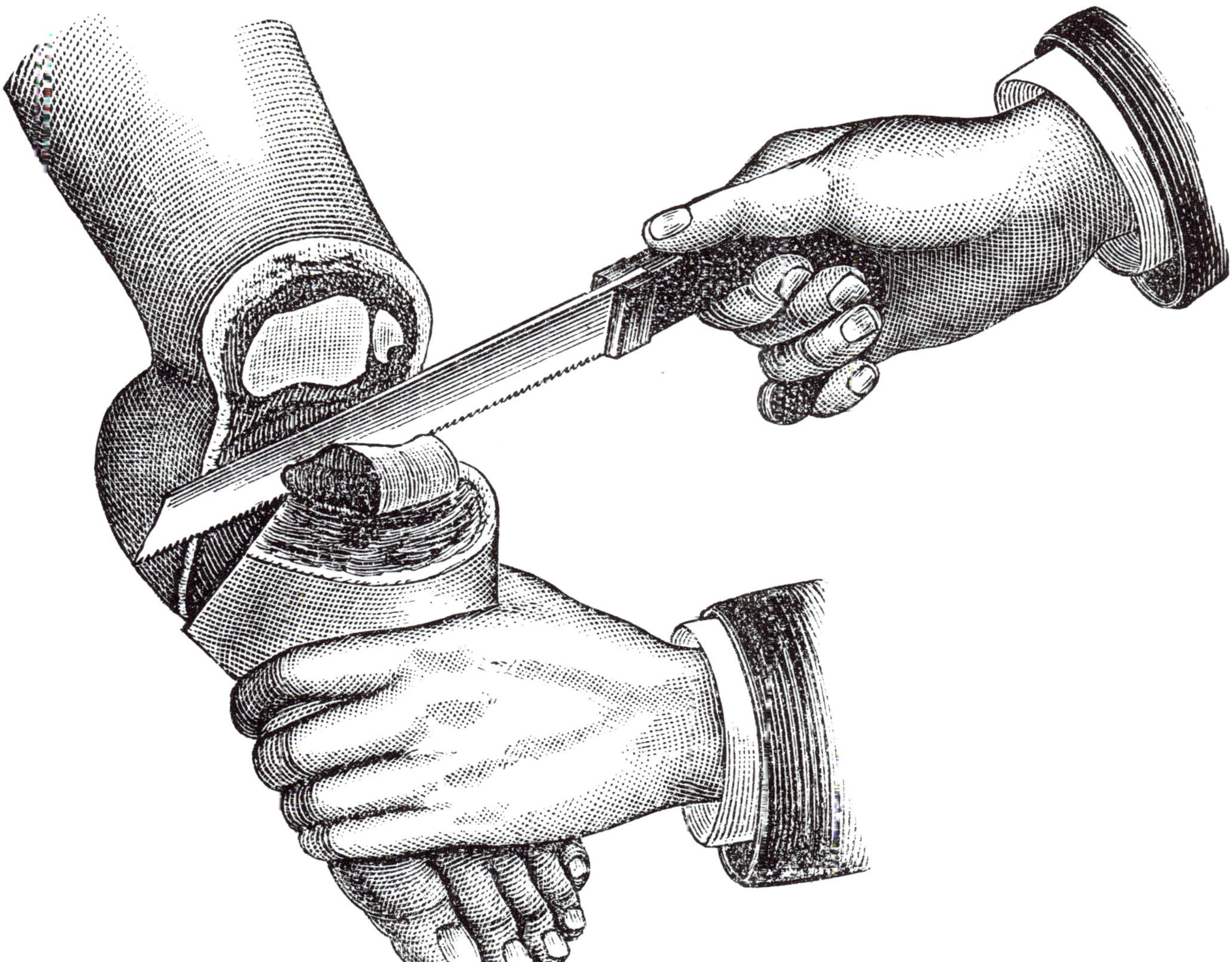

DISARTICULATION OF THE SECOND JOINT

The advantage of this operation is that it can be effected quickly and with no major complication.
It is quite common in view of labour accidents.

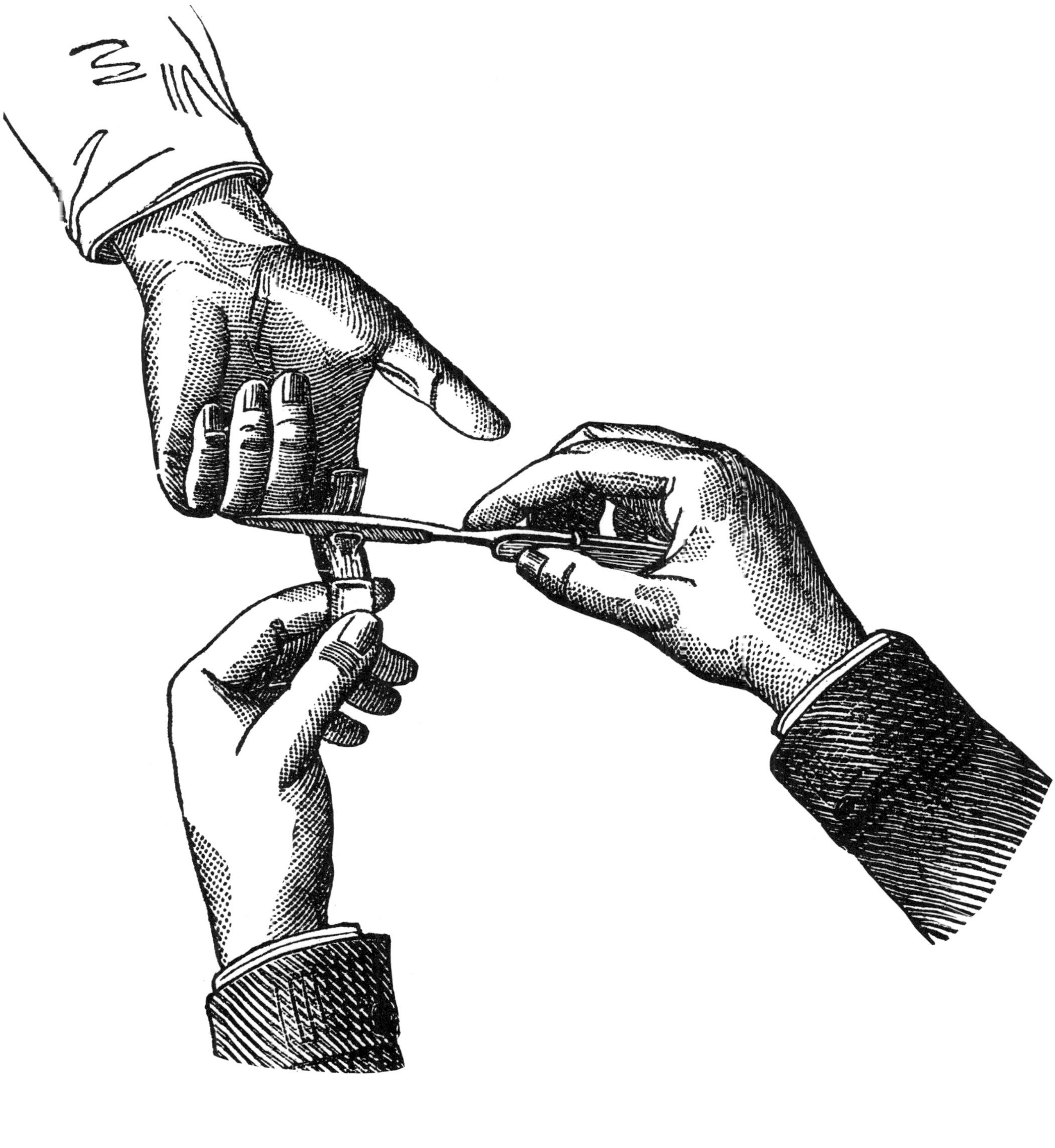

GORY PARTURITION

If the child dies prematurely, he is cut up before removal to avoid injury to the patient. The pieces are removed one by one and reassembled to make sure that nothing has been forgotten in the uterus.

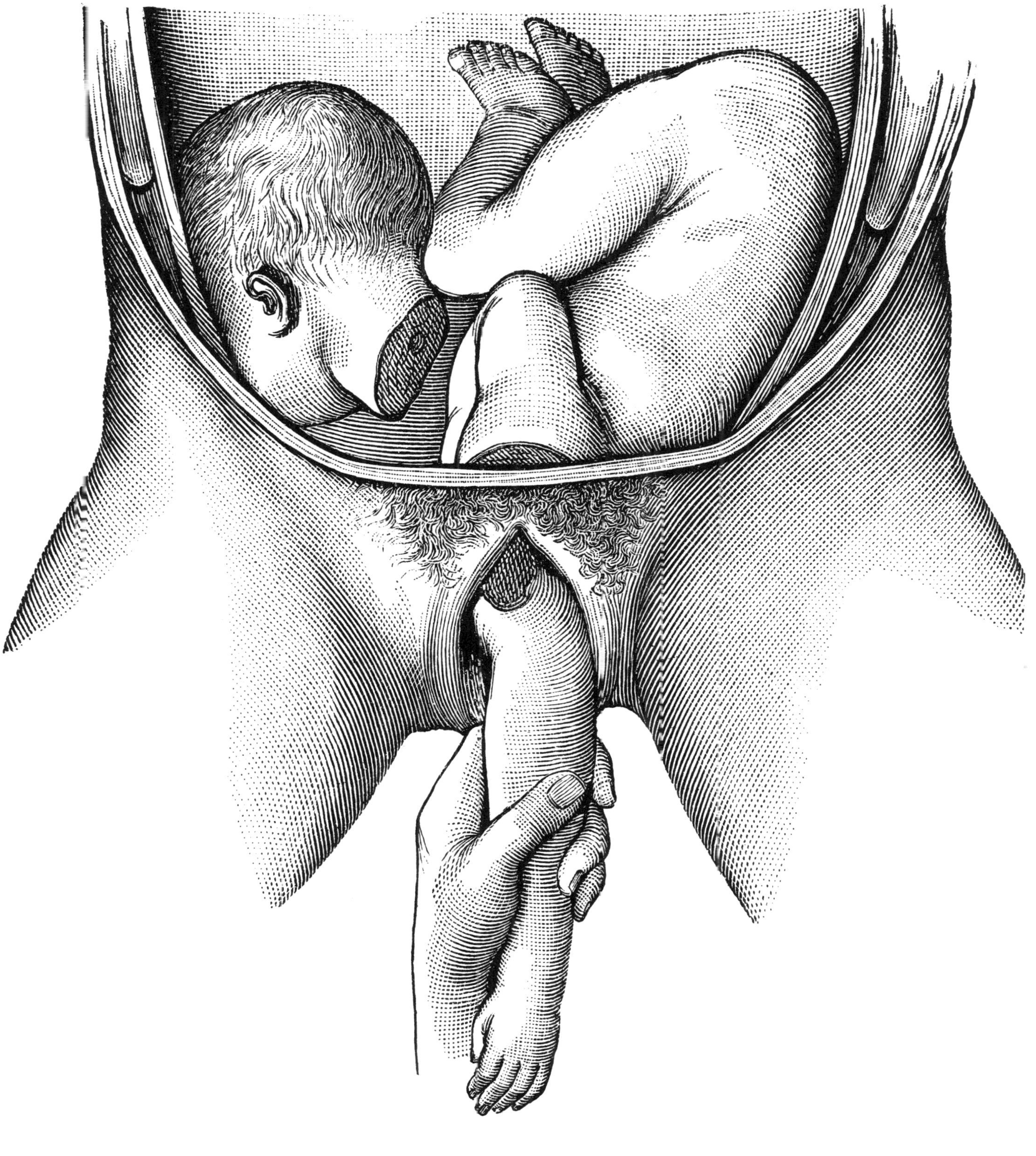

SOUNDING A CALCULUS BY PERCUSSION

Once the stone is formed in the bladder it never dissolves of its own accord. Aside from lithotomy, which consists of cutting into the bladder, either through the lower abdomen or through the perineum, there is the system of lithotrity, which consists of approaching the bladder stone through natural passages and of grinding it into pieces more easy to discharge.

One method is to abrade the stone from its periphery toward the centre, but this is more theoretical than practical, as none of the apparatus so far invented has yet been able to function properly on a living being.

One current generally applied method consists of directly squashing the stones, either by pressure or by percussion. Seated to the patient's right, the surgeon holds the device, the jaws of which have seized the stone in the bladder, in his left hand, and, armed with the hammer in his right hand, he proceeds to deliver sharp little blows.

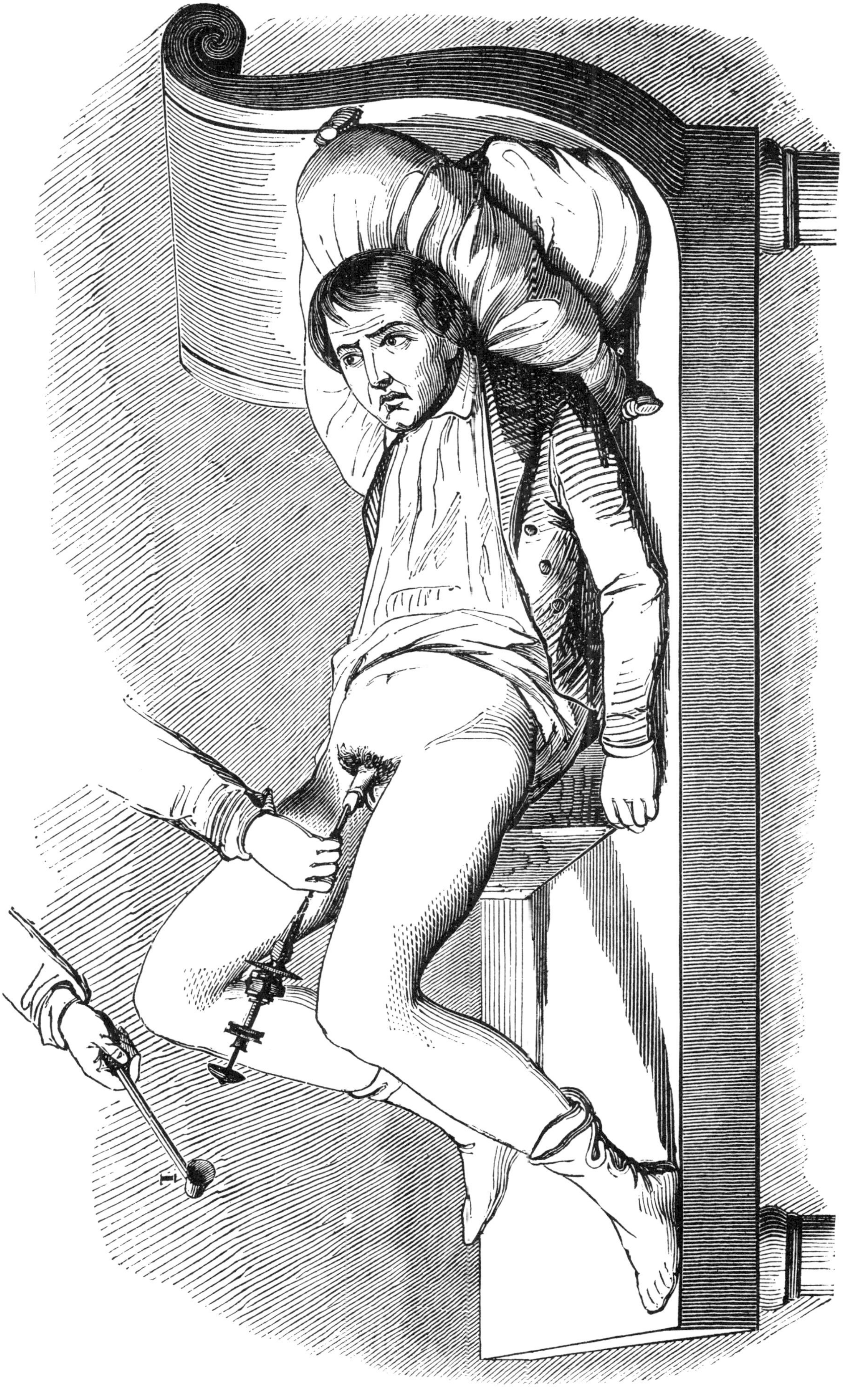

HYDRO ELECTROTHERAPIA

AQUATIC CRUTCH

Swimming is considered to afford excellent possibilities for muscular re-education. This brilliant aquatic support provides for both preparation to swimming and even for the practice of the latest waterless swimming.

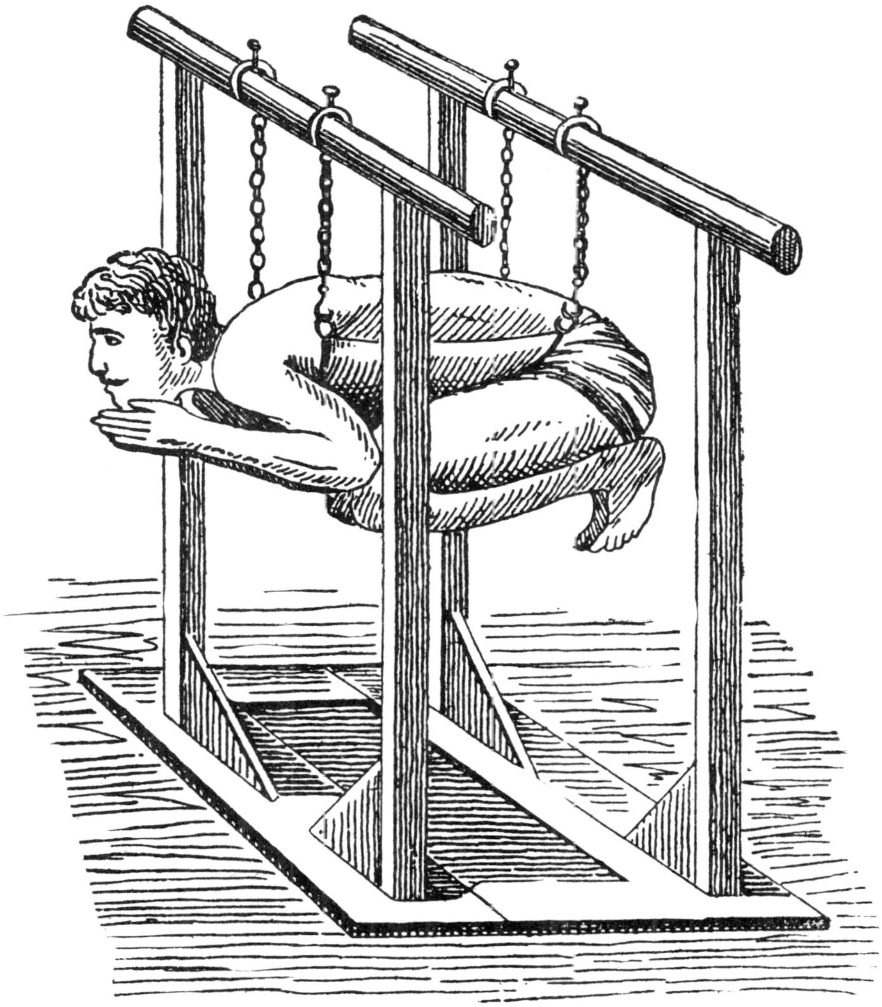

TREATMENT WITH WATER JET

The cold water jet is considered to be a tonic stimulant; it accelerates exchanges, stimulates organic functions, vivifies, and warms by reaction. So as to accelerate blood circulation in the lower abdomen and along the legs, the servant squirts very cool water, with slight circular motions.

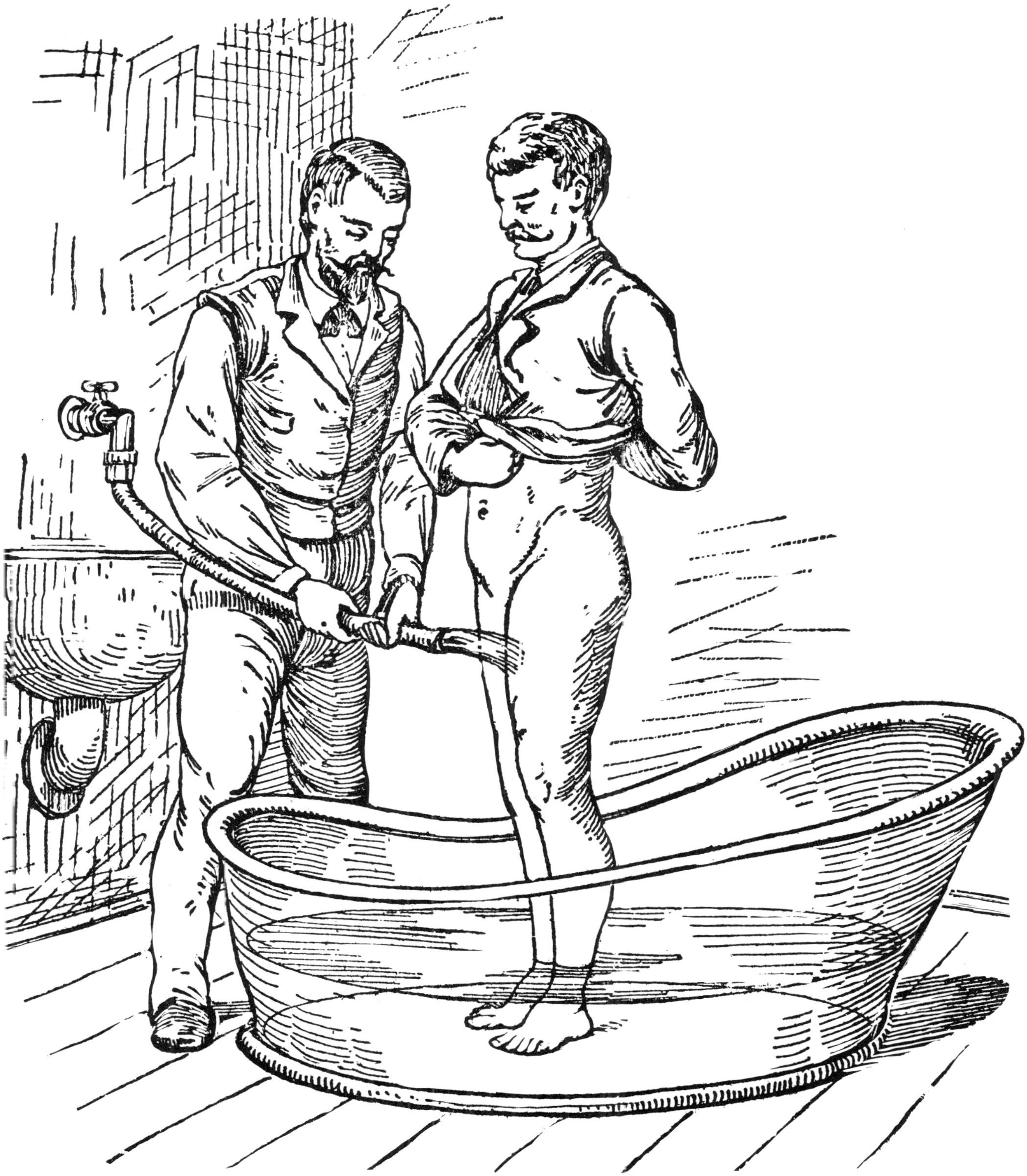

SWINGING BATH

This very recent model of an interior zinc bath-tub is an invitation to perform one's ablutions. It presents the advantages of five sorts of bath: complete bath, children's bath, sitz-bath, steam bath and agitated bath that refreshes and fortifies the nerves.

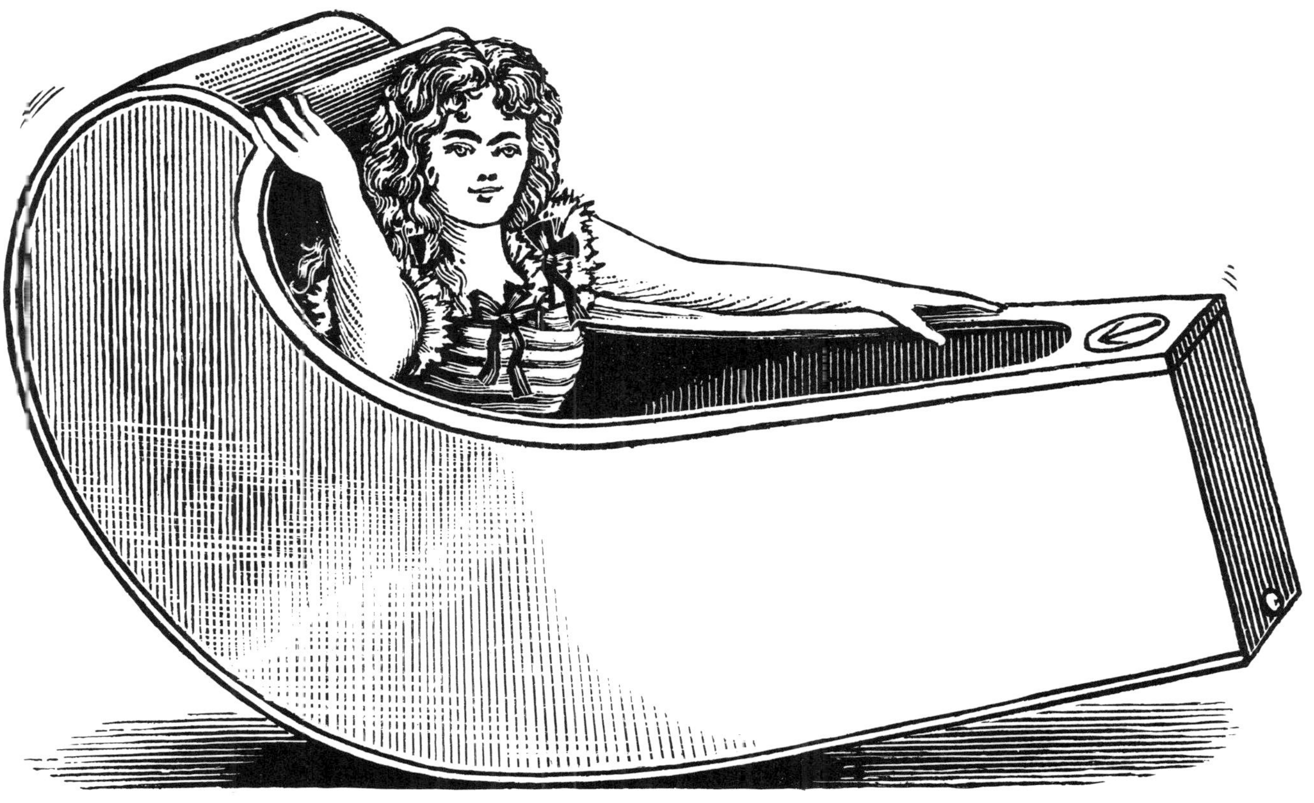

RECLINING STEAM BATH

The recumbent position is particularly indicated for those patients whose general state of health does not tolerate the sitting position.

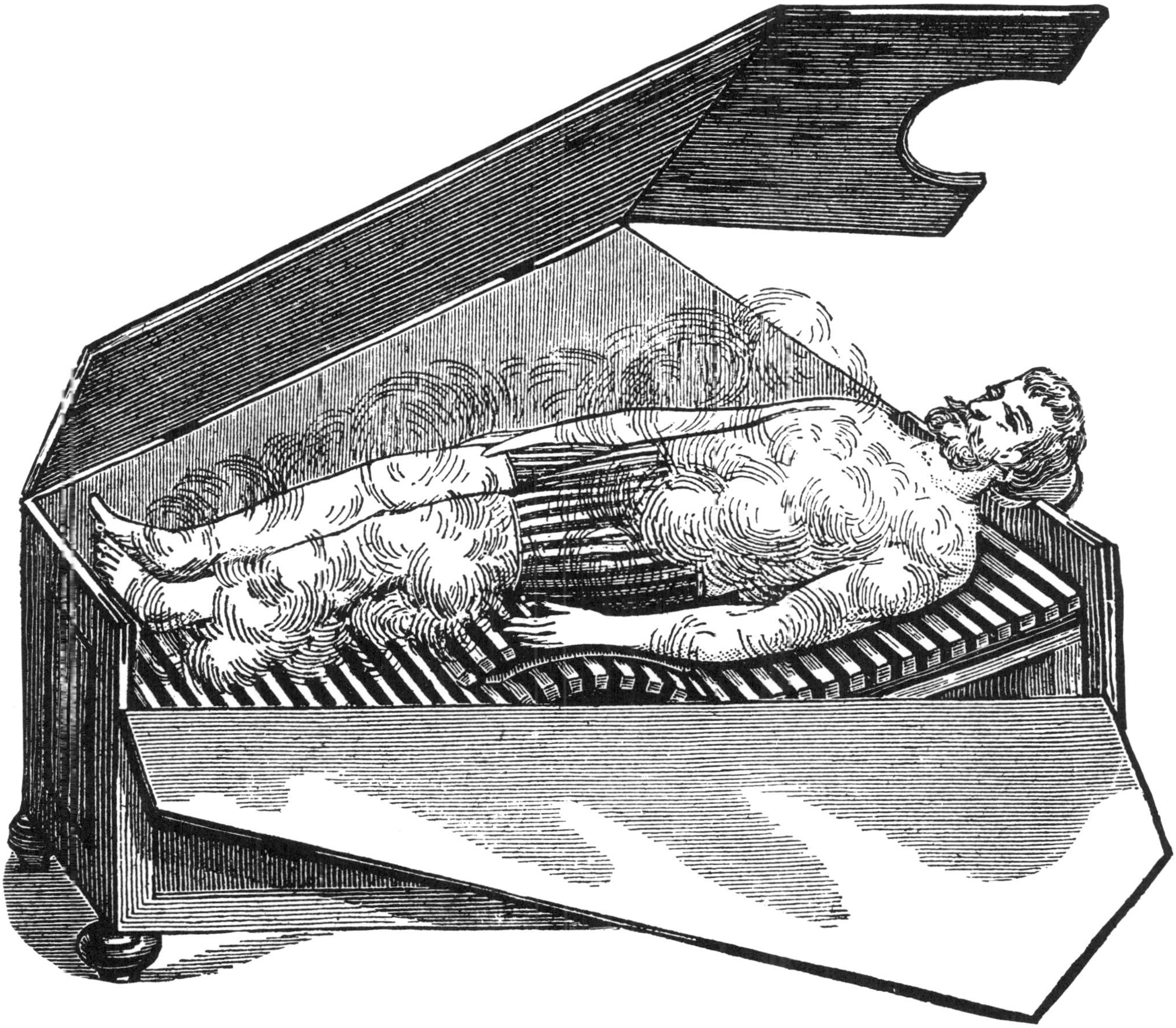

HOT AIR BATH

Patients derive the greatest of benefits from complete hot air baths, taken lying down, the head remaining in fresh air. They induce perspiration without overexertion. One should generally not go beyond the temperatures of seventy to eighty degrees centigrade.

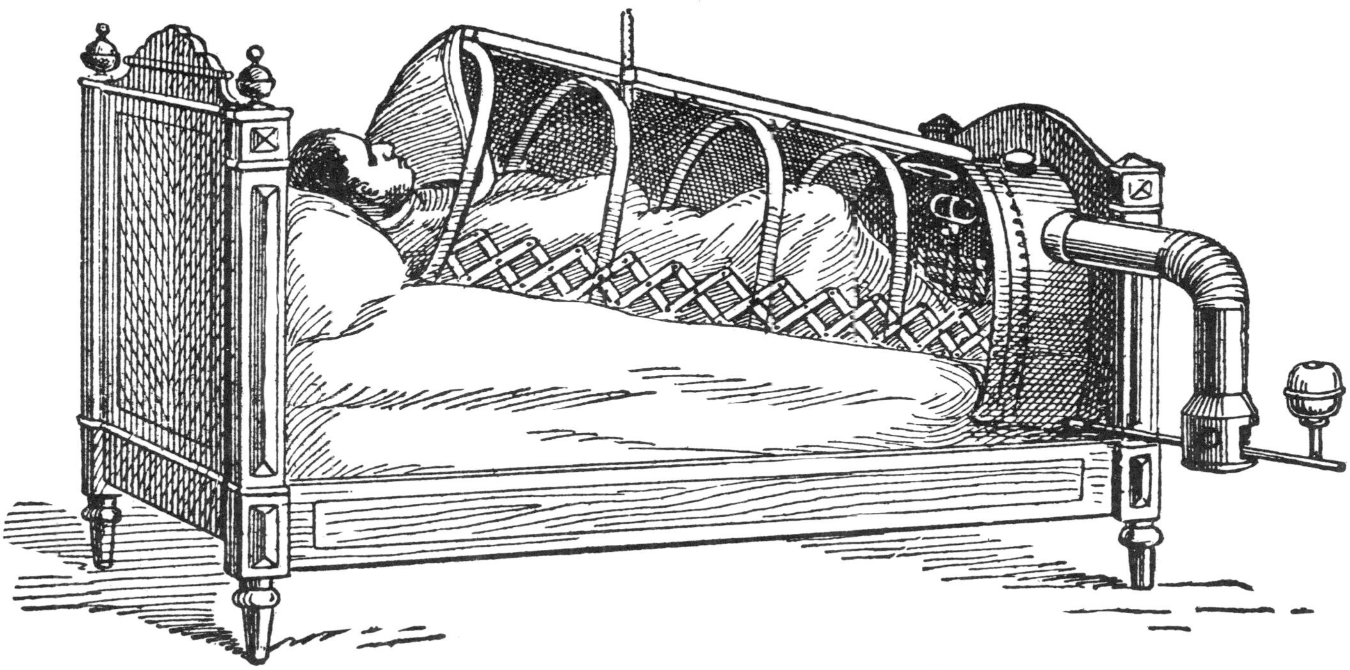

PARTITIONED ELECTRIC BATH

This type of bath-tub allows one to use the therapeutic effects of cataphoresis, by impregnating the body with iron, mercury and lithium by a judicious anode-cathode wiring and the dilution of chemical solutions.

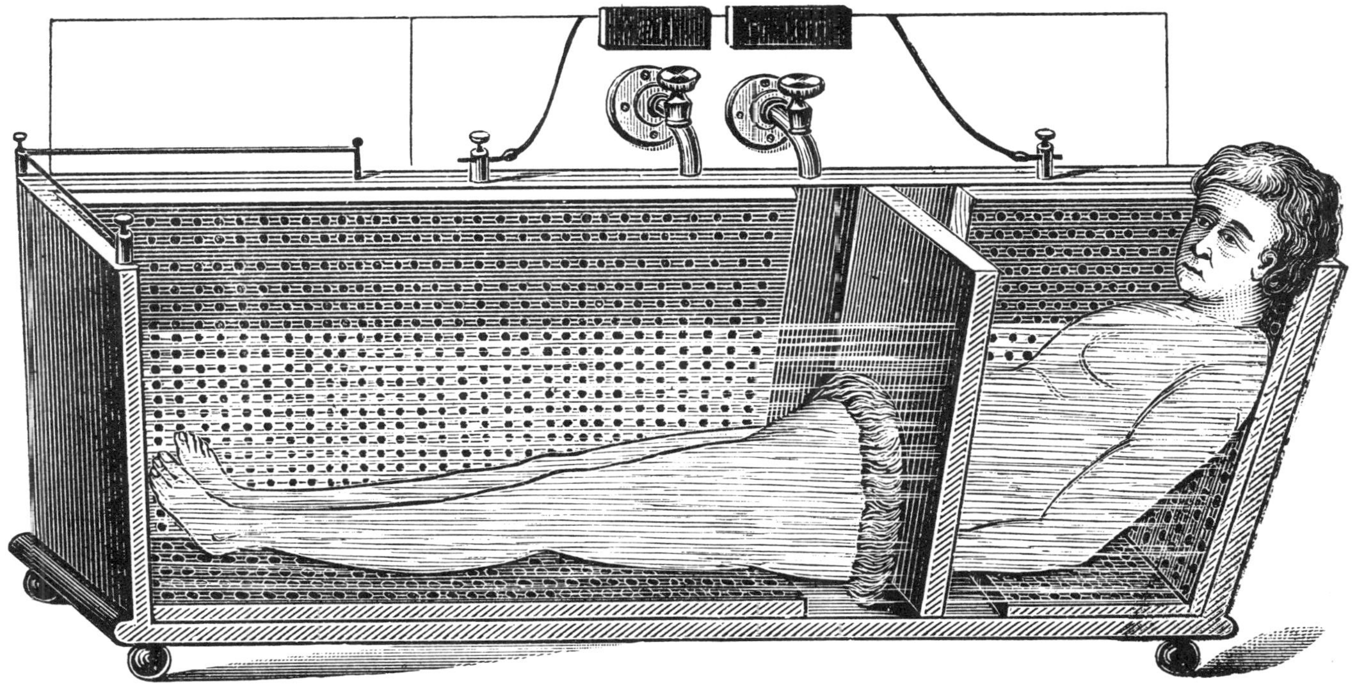

WATER CIRCULATION

In the case of nervous dyspepsia or in cardialgia, the water is sent through a circular pipe. The bath lasts for one hour, and a towel is disposed so as to protect against possible burns. In the case of dyspepsia accompanied by tenacious vomiting, meals should be taken during the treatment.

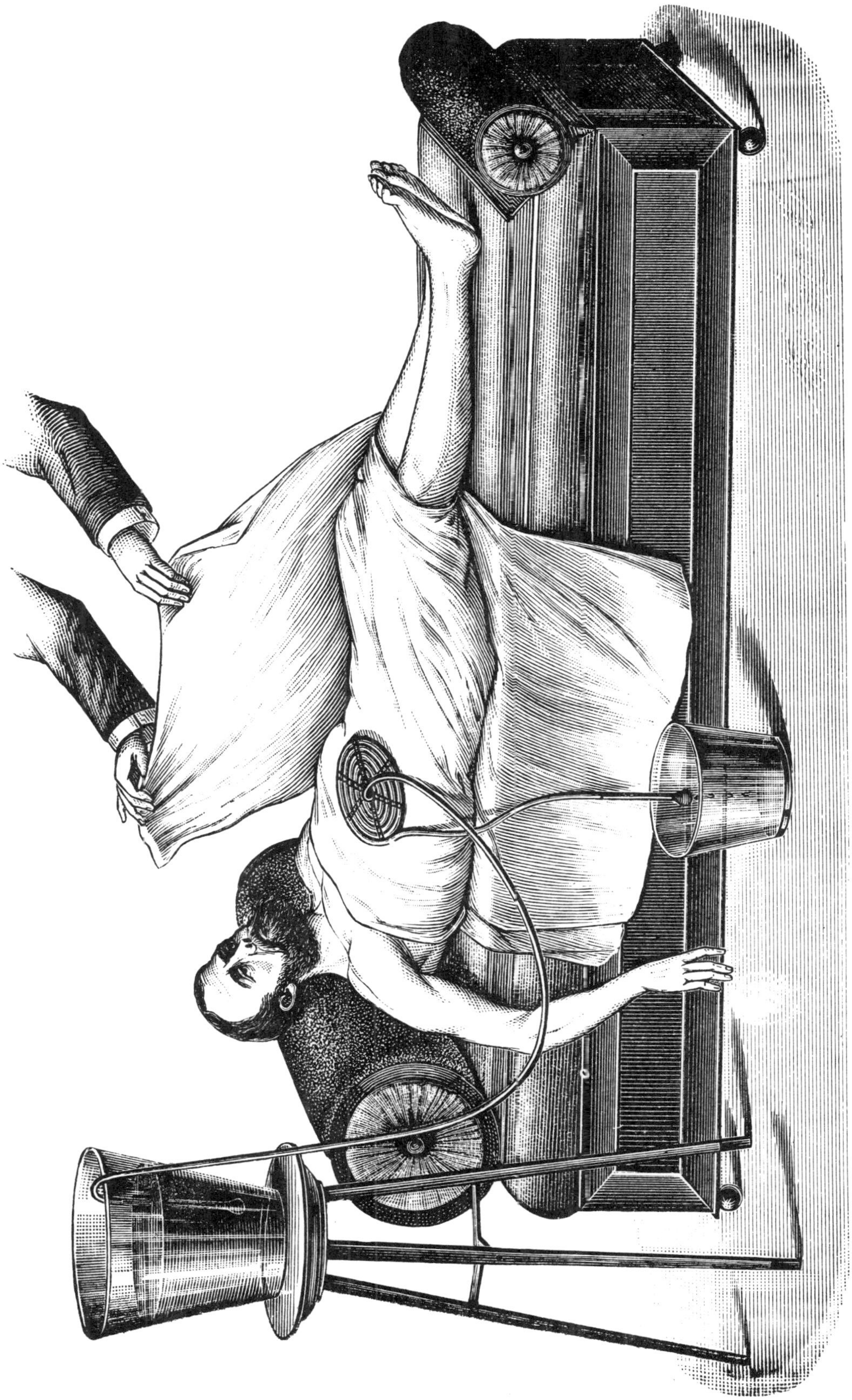

FRANKLINISATION

Franklinisation or static electricity is therapeutically indicated for neurasthenia, migraine and hysteria. The patient, placed on an insulating podium, immediately feels, once the apparatus begins to function, a sensation comparable to that of a gauze veil lightly brushing against his face.
A sudden discharge resulting in a spark that lends a certain pallor to the teguments may be caused by holding a metallic ball near to the patient. In the case of the muscles, quite energetic tremors and contractions in proportion to the length of the sparks can be observed.

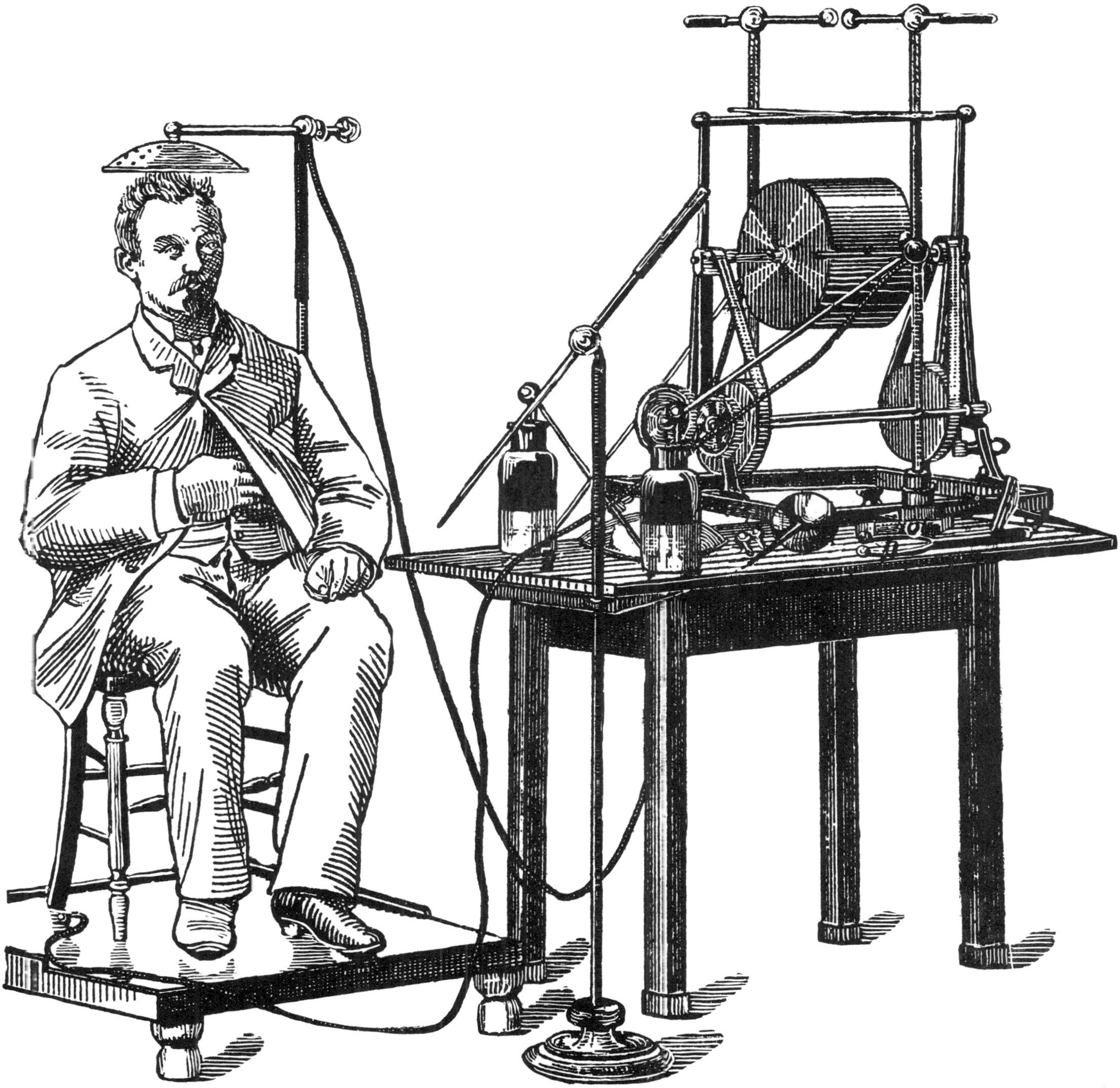

MECANOTHERAPIA

AMERICAN DRESSING FOR FRACTURED THIGHS

This American dressing is a continuous traction device that necessitates tensile stress on the limb and that subsequently leads to stiffness of the knee. It is possible, when using the American dressing, to lessen the effects of prolonged extension by giving very slight daily exercise to the knee after the twentieth day, without disturbing the dressing.

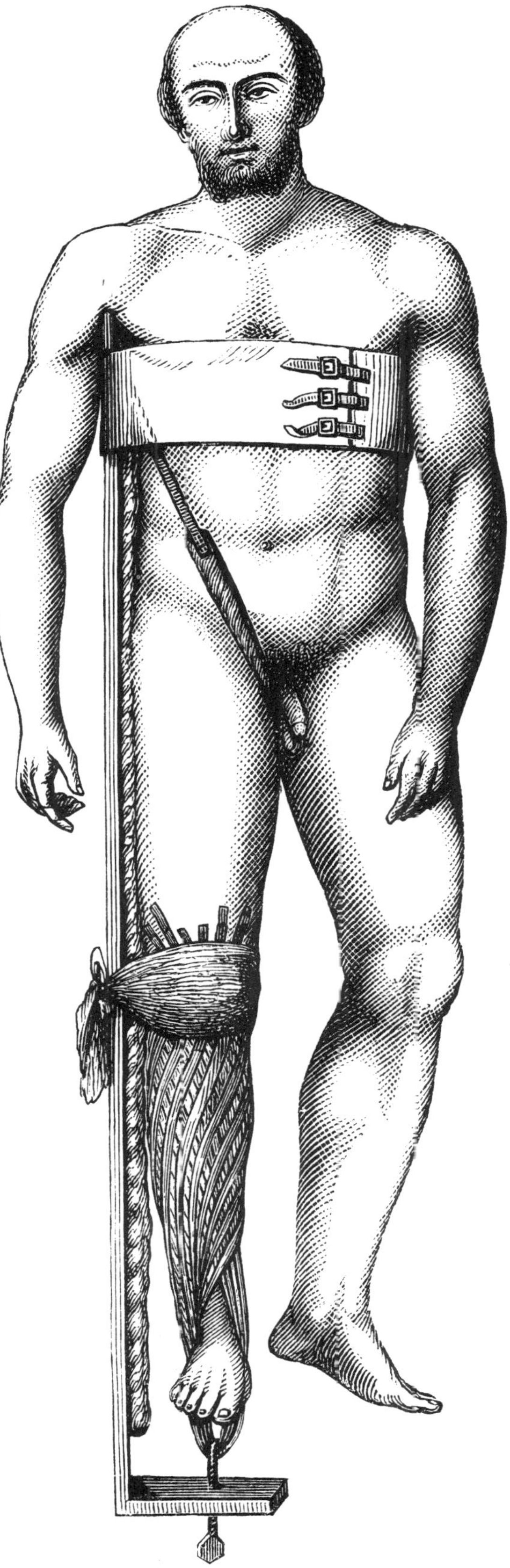

SETTING A DISLOCATED SHOULDER

The patient is seated on a chair. The first assistant slips a sheet or towel folded as a scarf under the dislocated arm. The second assistant wraps the lower end of the dislocated arm with a compress or even with a wet handkerchief, and grasps the arm with both hands just above the elbow.

Then both assistants lean backwards and exert traction in opposite directions on all the muscles of the arm and shoulder.

By the third minute the assistants are tired, and their fatigue can be ascertained by the state of congestion of their hands that are purplish-blue. At this point they must be relayed one by one, taking care that the traction is not interrupted in the process. The surgeon, in the meantime, follows the progress of the apophysis of the humerus under the armpit. During a few seconds, the patient complains and says: I can't stand it. He can be seen to be weakening, and at that precise moment the dislocation is reduced. This generally occurs at the eighth minute, sometimes noisily, sometimes quietly.

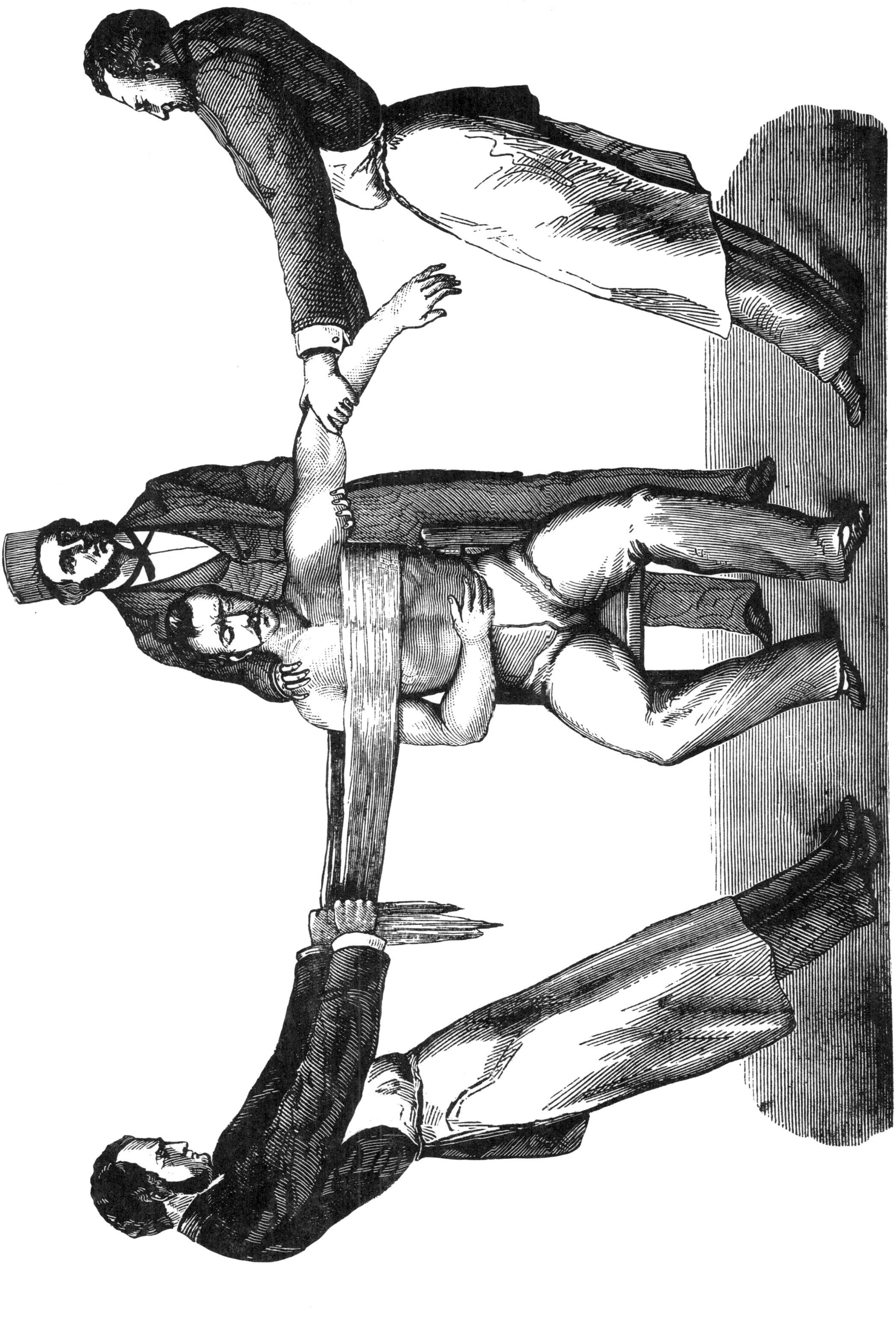

UPRIGHT BED

Phelps' "upright bed" allows the spinal column to be at rest while adjusting with precision the degree of extension necessary to correct its gibbousness.

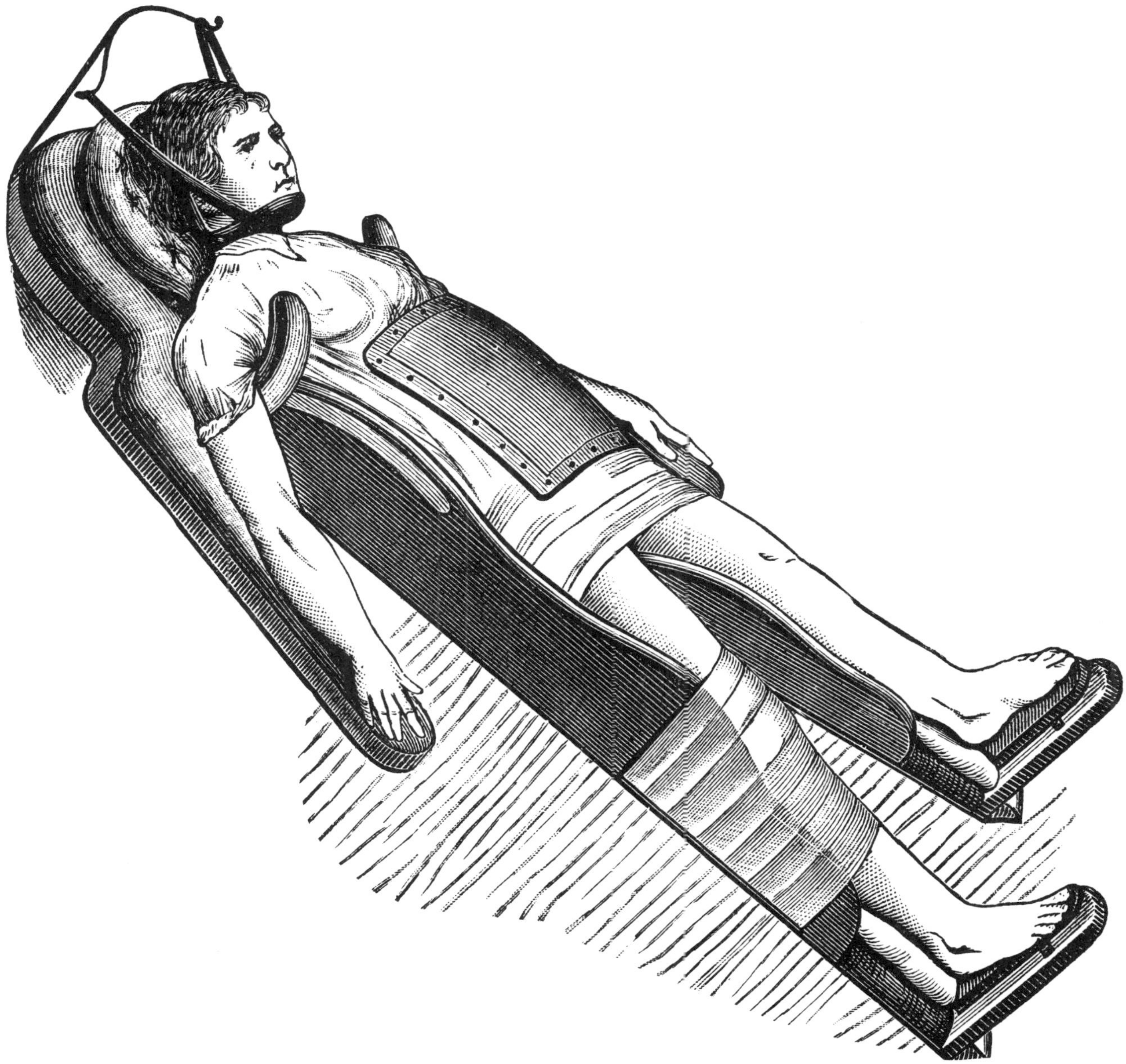

CANTING COLLAR

For the treatment of a stiff neck, metallic collars are highly effective. They are heavily constructed and they either hinder the neck or communicate to it the movements of the body. This device has the advantage of not exercising circular compression around the head and of leaving the neck free.

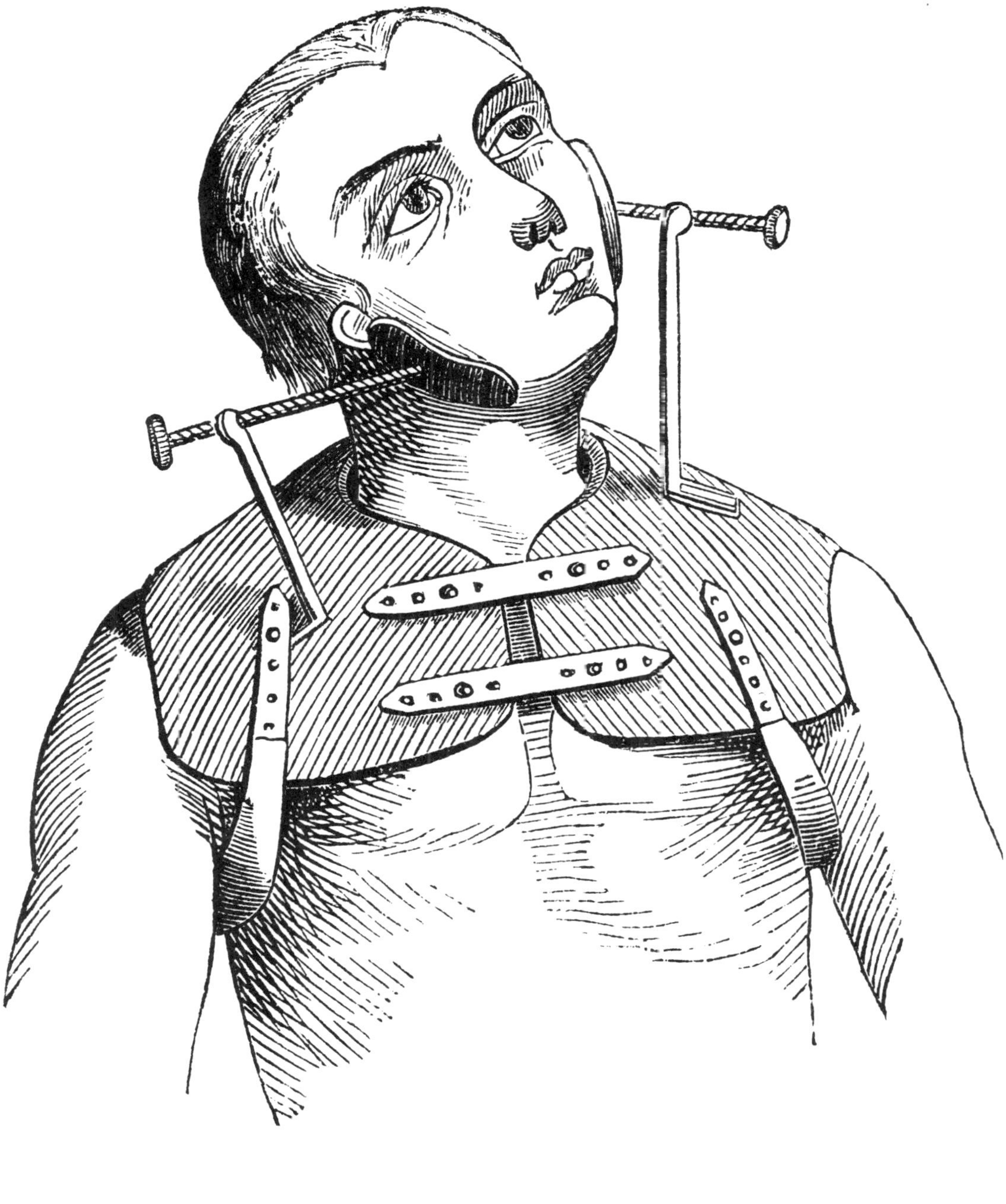

MECHANOTHERAPY FOR THE ARMS

The patient is placed on an adjustable seat. Thanks to two previously adjusted handles, he moves two rods around an axle causing the weights to pivot. This active mechanotherapy is particularly successful for re-educating the arms.

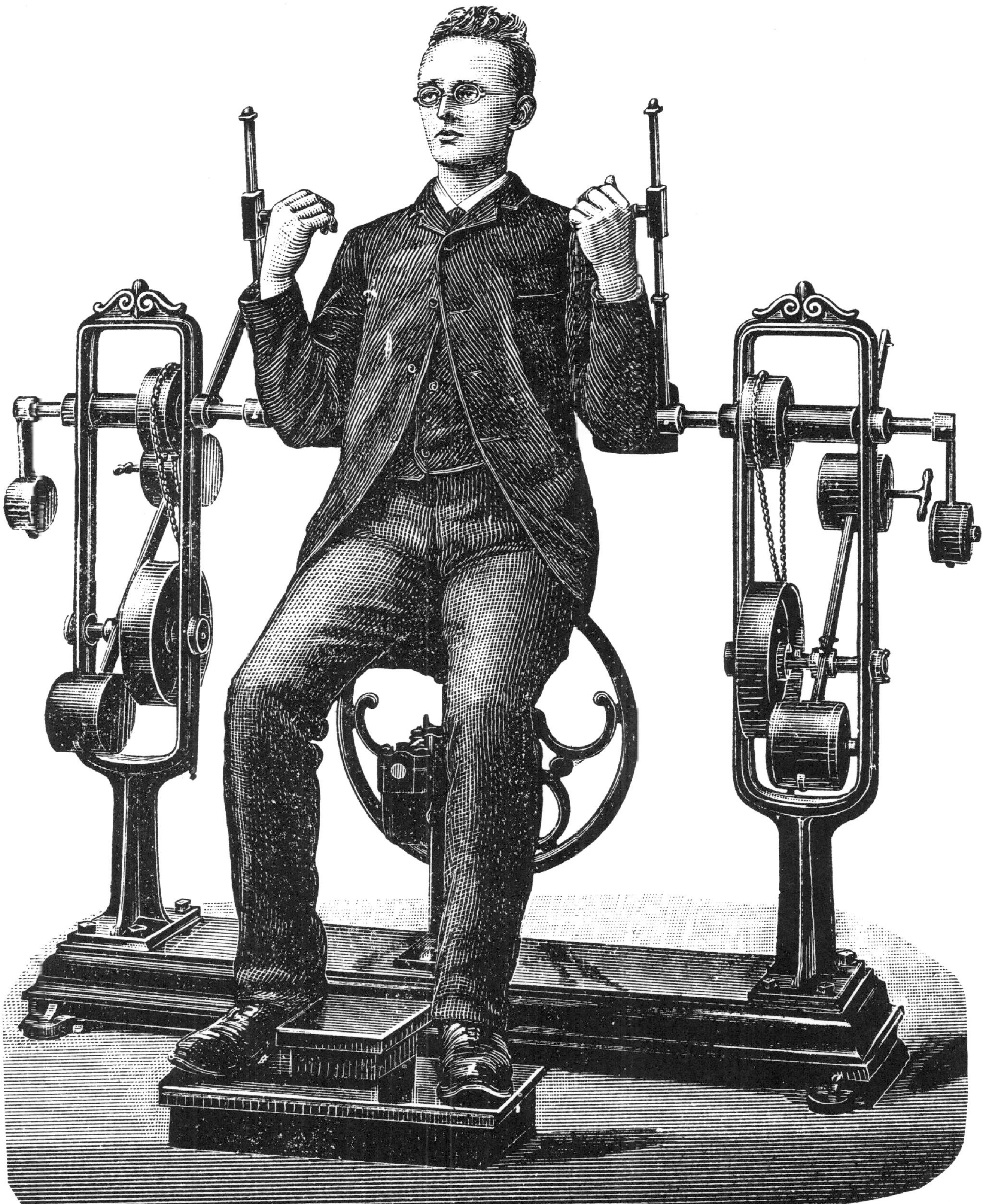

MECHANOTHERAPY FOR THE BACK

In this case it is a question of passive mechanotherapy. This ingenious apparatus mechanically massages the dorsal region.

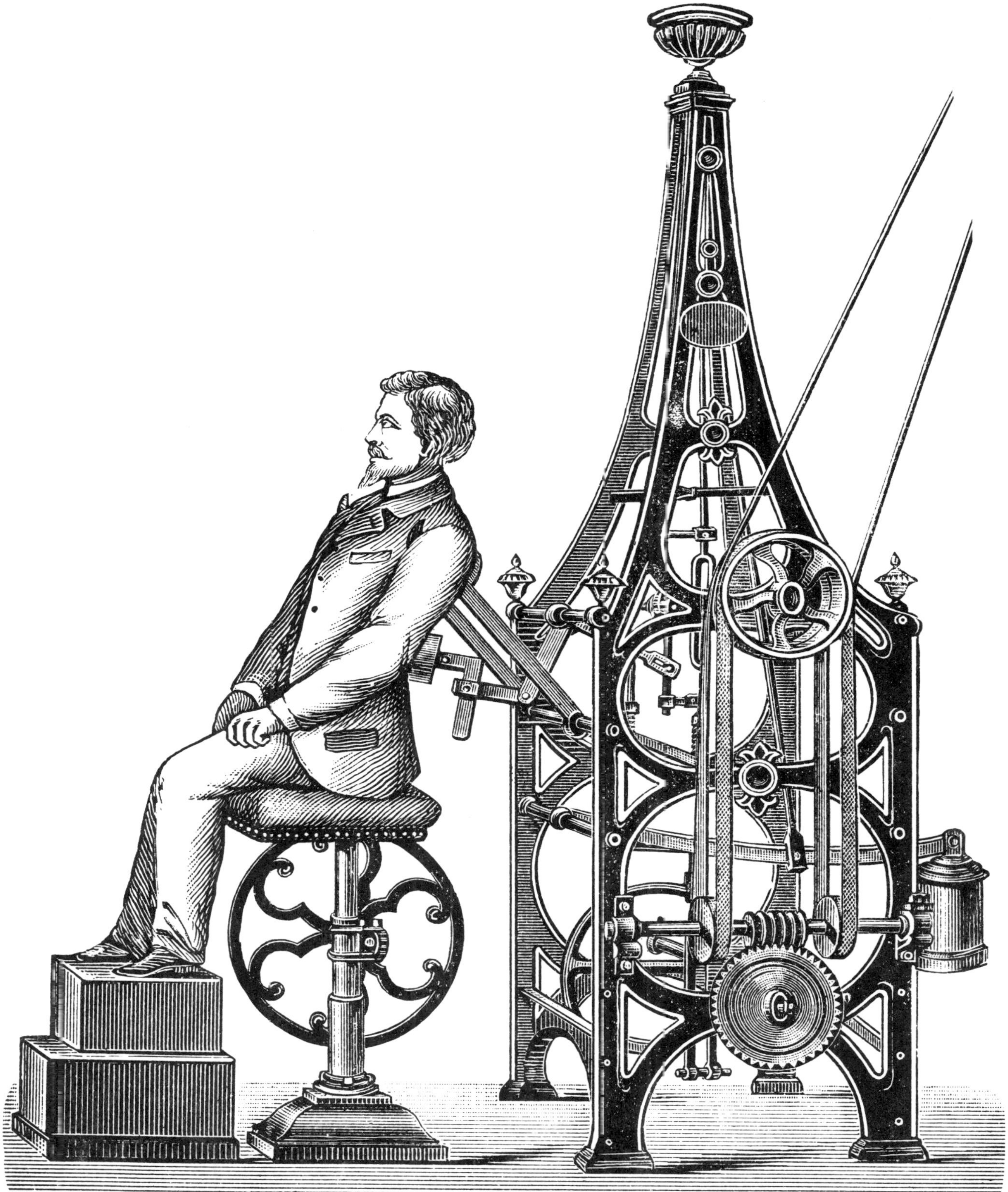

MECHANOTHERAPY FOR THE LEGS

This impressive mechanism, composed of a cupboard armed with supports, cross-pieces and various appurtenances, is helpful in an active mechanotherapy for the lower limbs.

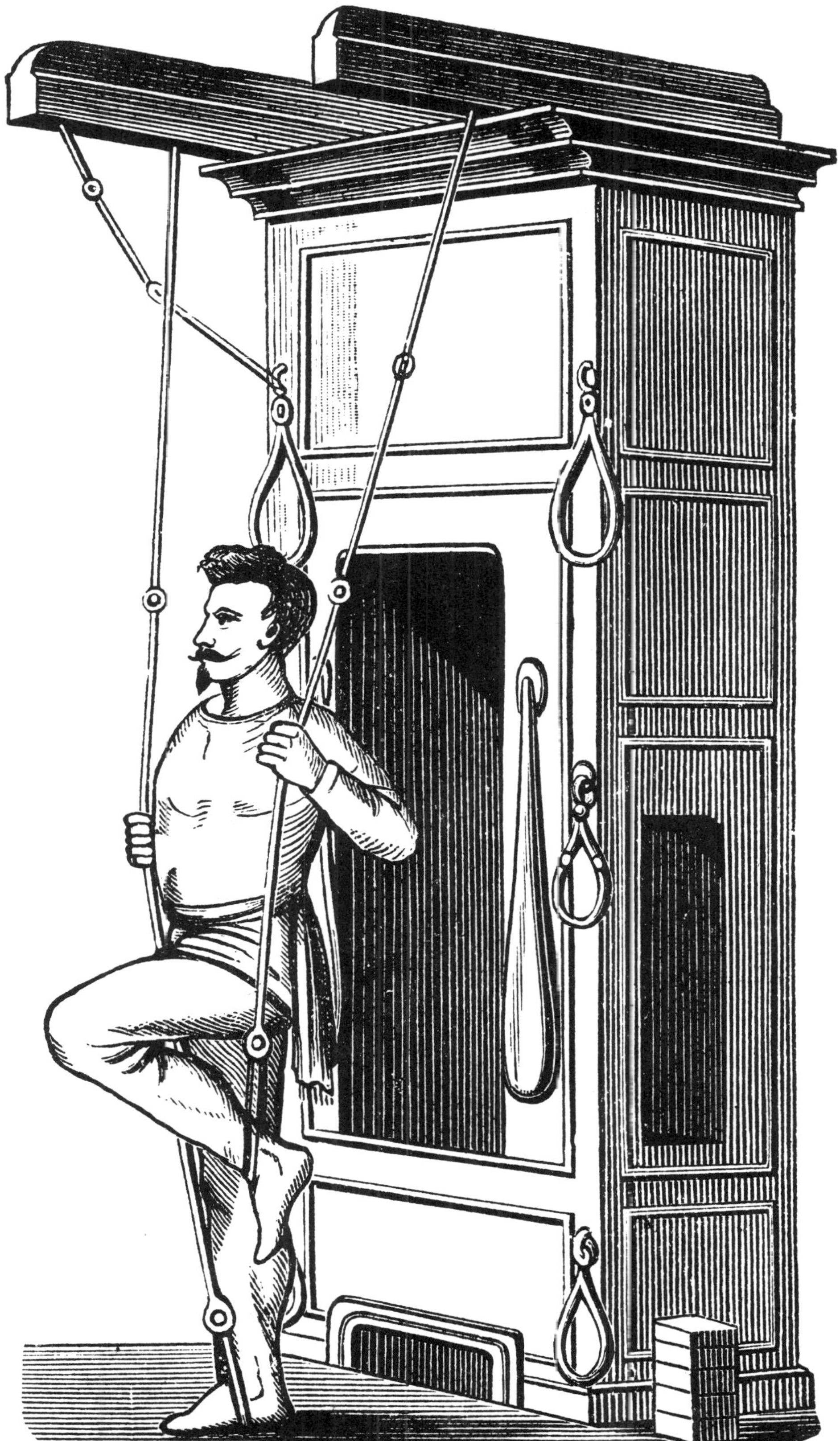

MECHANOTHERAPY FOR THE LEGS

Thanks to ropes, weights and a sort of yoke, the patient performs limbering and re-educating exercises.

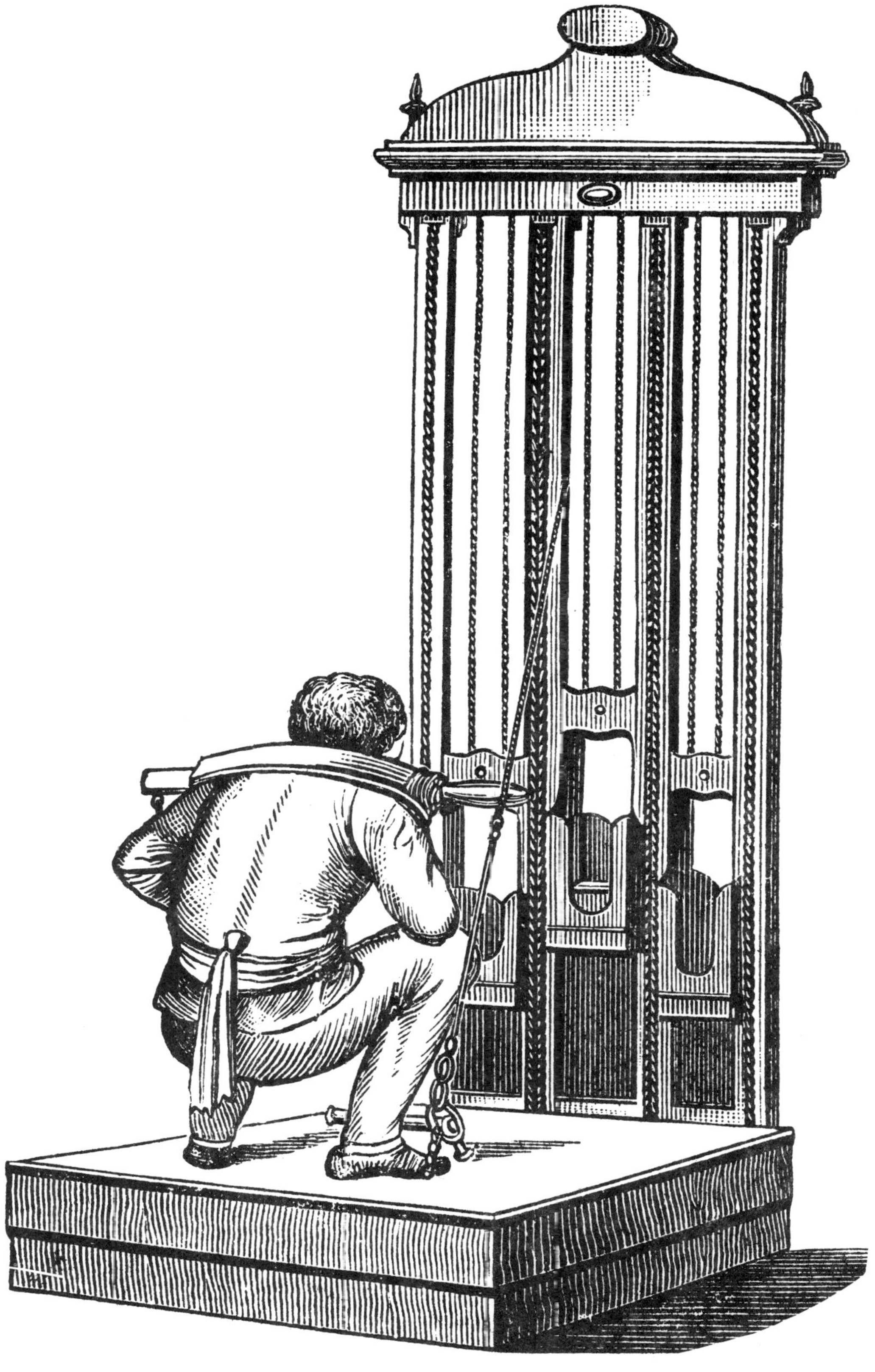

TREATMENT OF SCOLIOSIS

This method of lateral suspension is used in infantile orthopedy to correct scoliosis. The orthopodist presses vigorously on the girl's breast, which is very painful for the first few sessions. Later on, the girl becomes used to these manoeuvres.

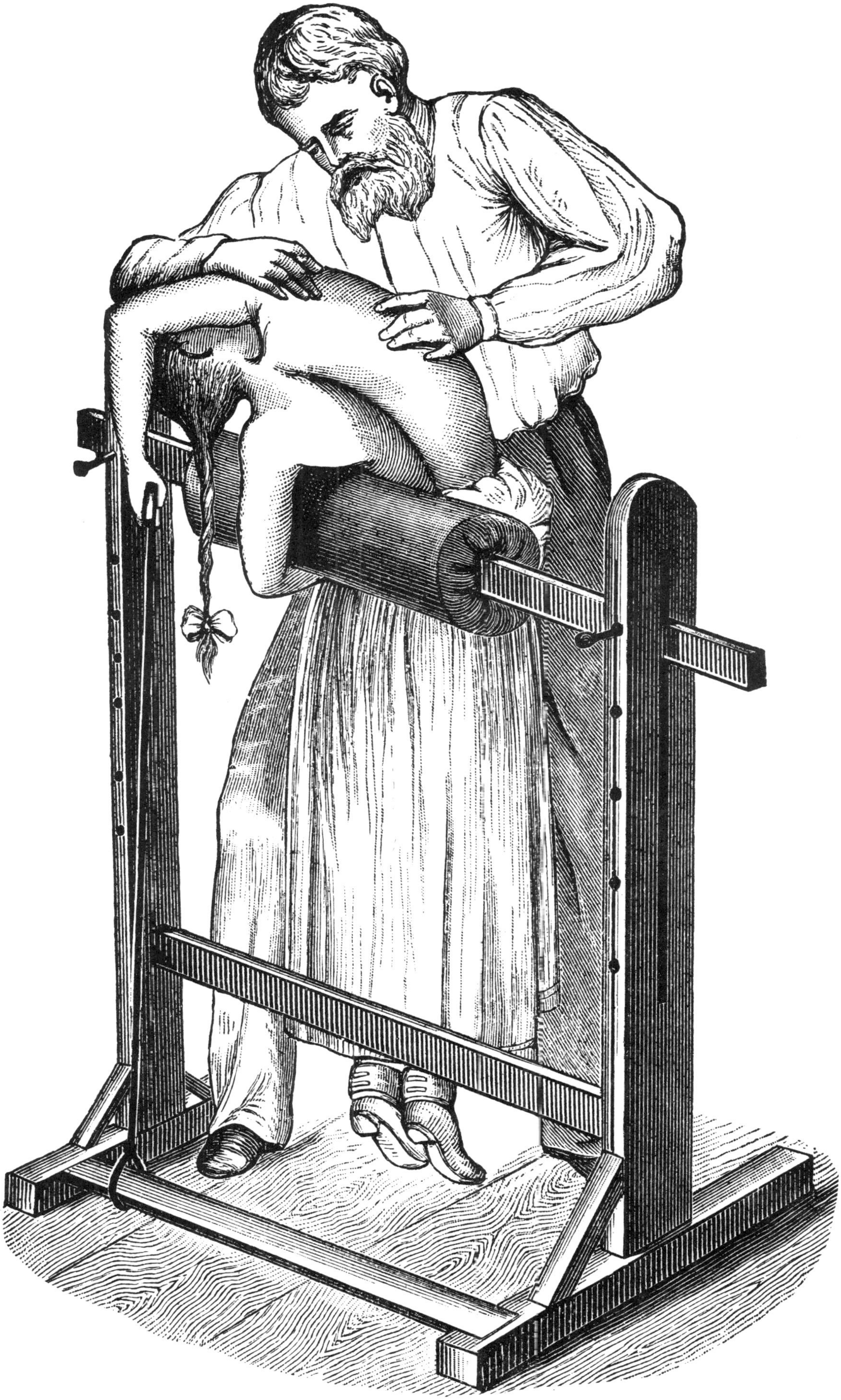

EXTENSION

The originality of this apparatus allows the young patient to adjust the intensity of the extension herself.

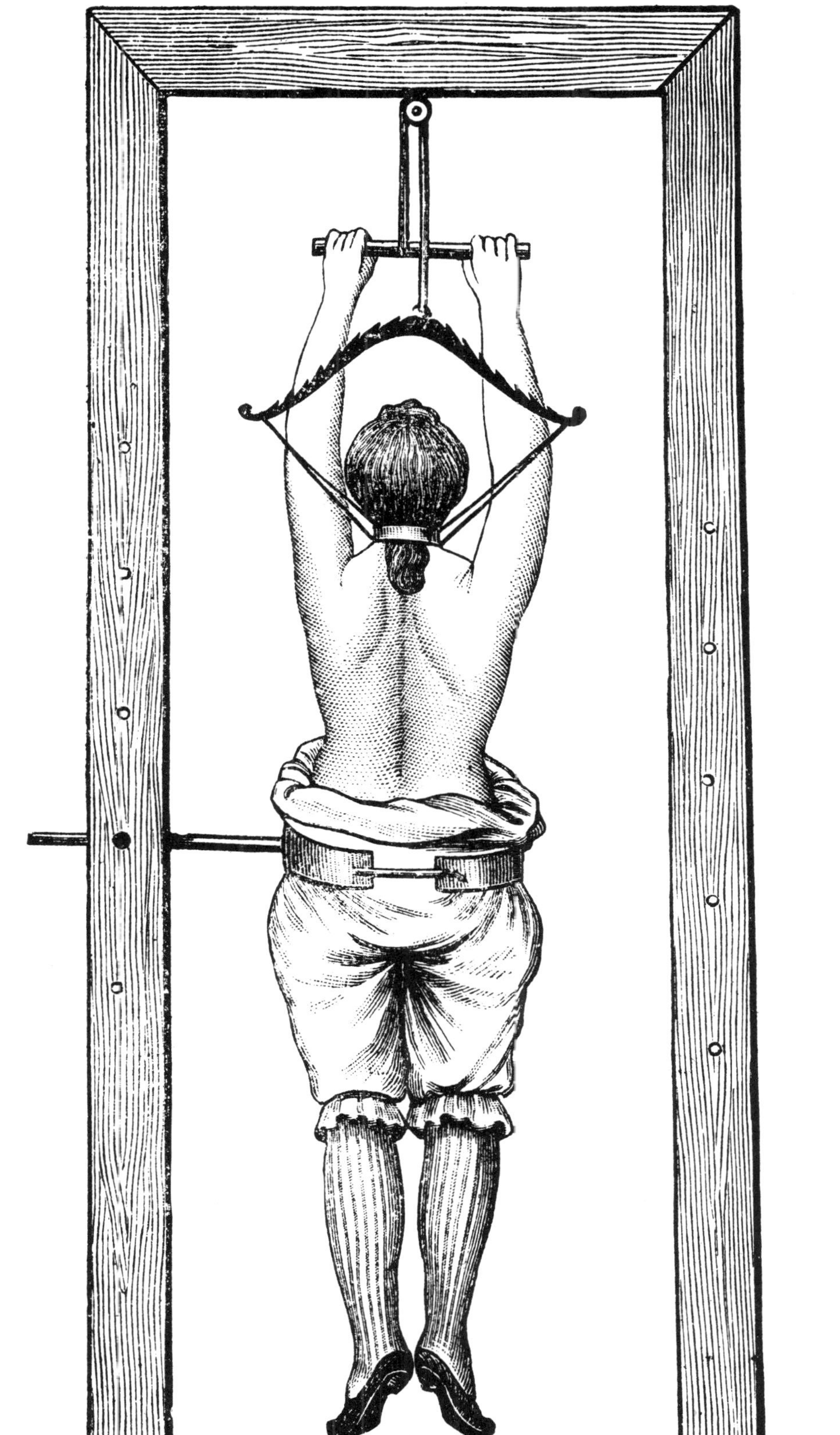

SUSPENSION WITH LATERAL COMPRESSION

This therapeutic process for medulla oblongata consists in suspending the patient a few centimetres from the ground thanks to a contrivance of straps supporting the chin, the nape of the neck, the armpits and the elbows. Sessions are repeated every two days, during six to eight weeks. The patient should be warned that any inopportune movement may be dangerous.

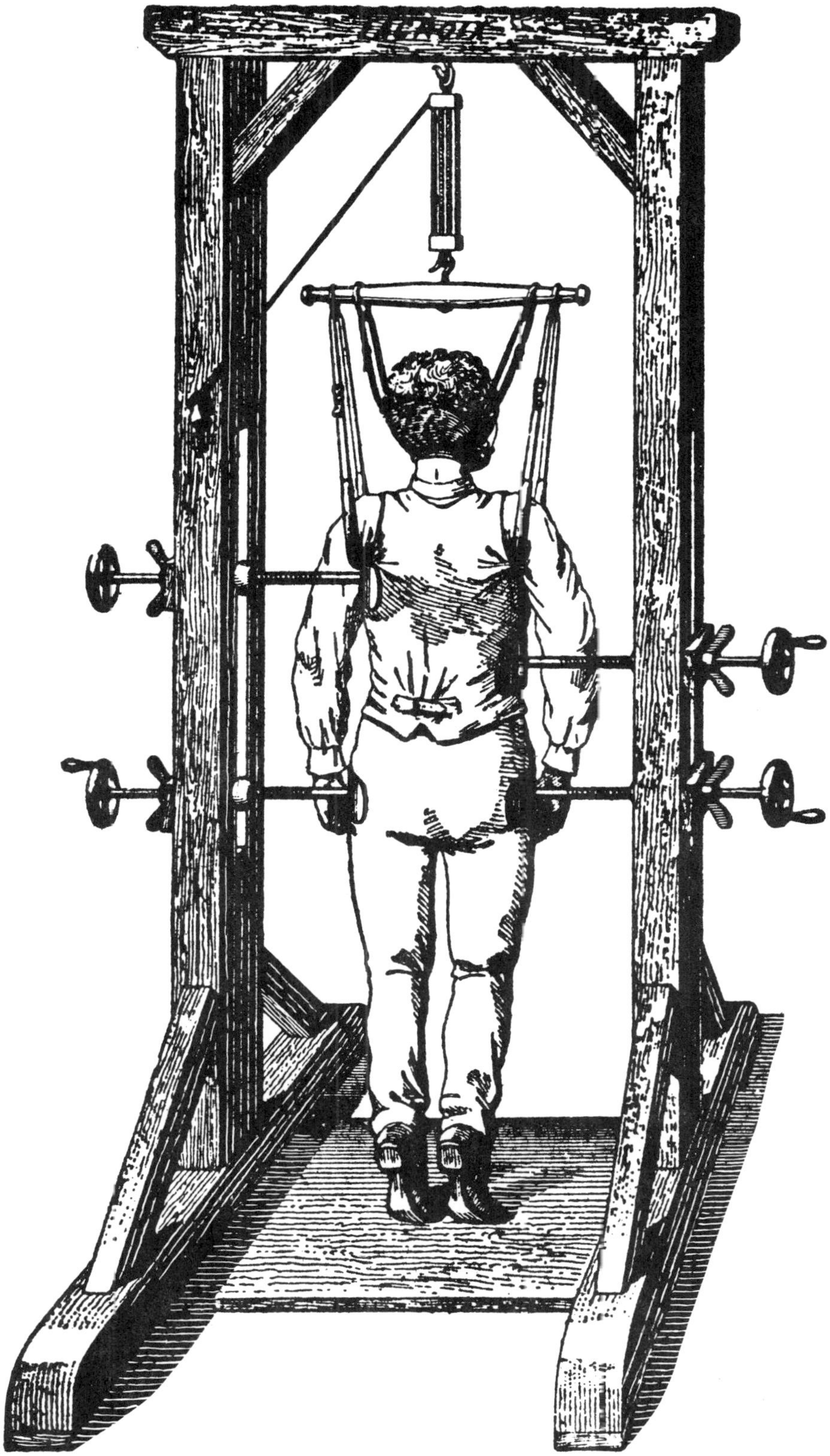

SUSPENSION

The particular interest of this suspension apparatus lies in the fact that it can be of use in treating nervous syphilis, bladder disorders and impotence.

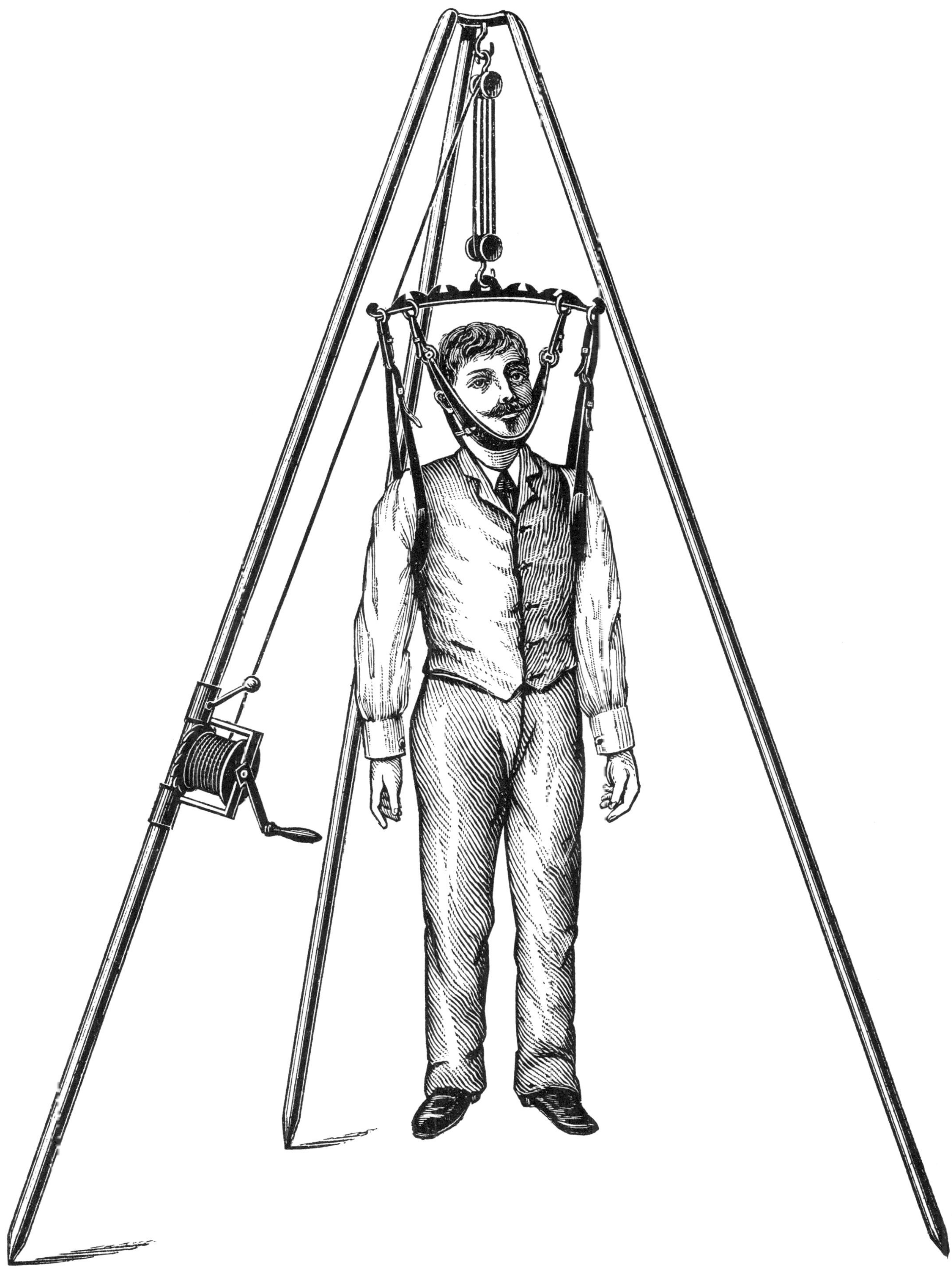

THORACOGRAPH

The thoracograph is an ingenious machine that gives a graphic representation of the chest, inhaling and exhaling, on a paper disc.

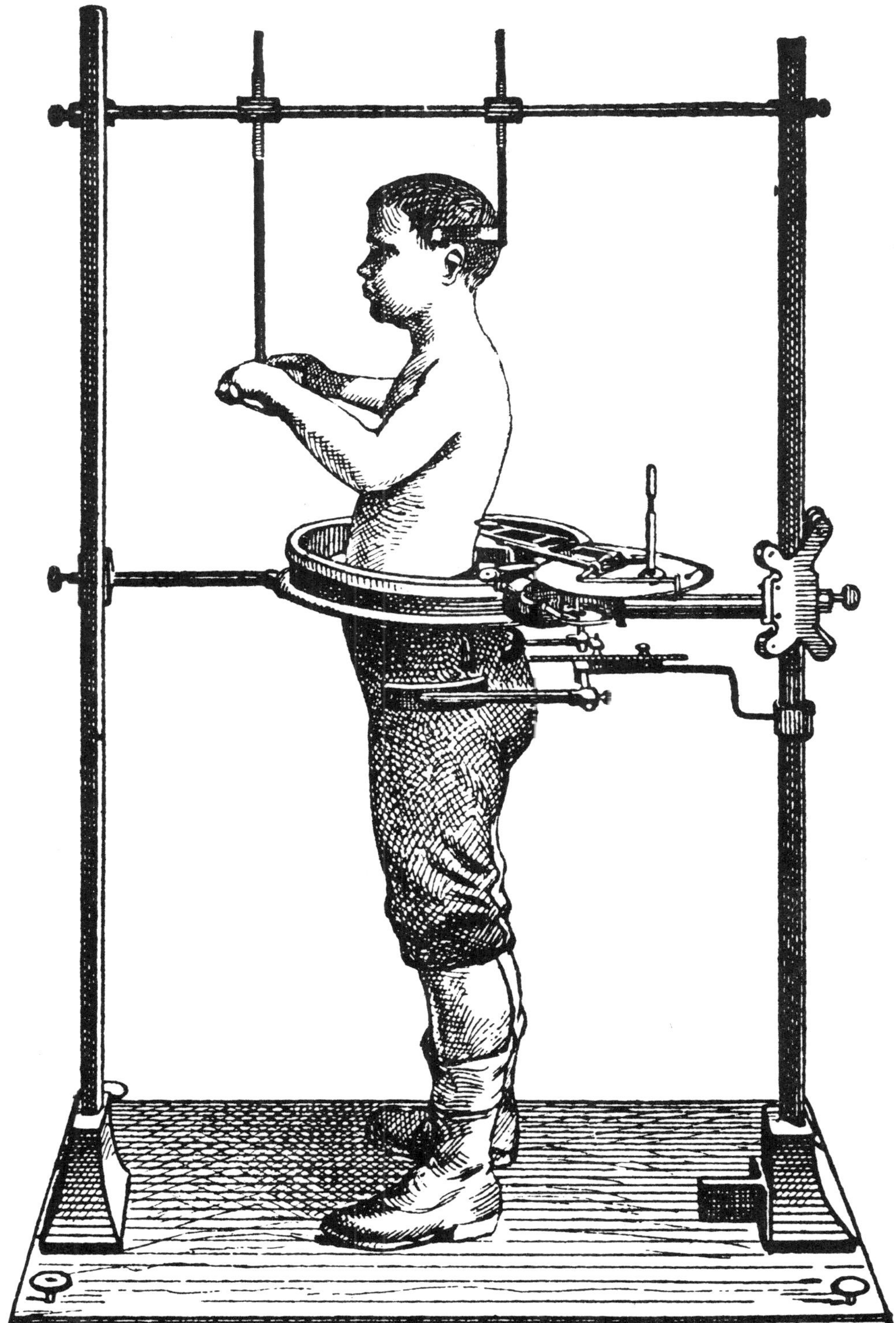

TERATOLOGIA

HETEROPAGIA

These are doubly parasitic monsters. In heteropagia, there is the fusion of two beings, one of which is so underdeveloped that he could not live independently from the one who carries him. The presence of a parasite suspended on the anterior face of the principal body is characteristic. If the heterotype parasite possesses a head and distinct limbs, the whole is termed heteropagia. This monstrosity is very rare.

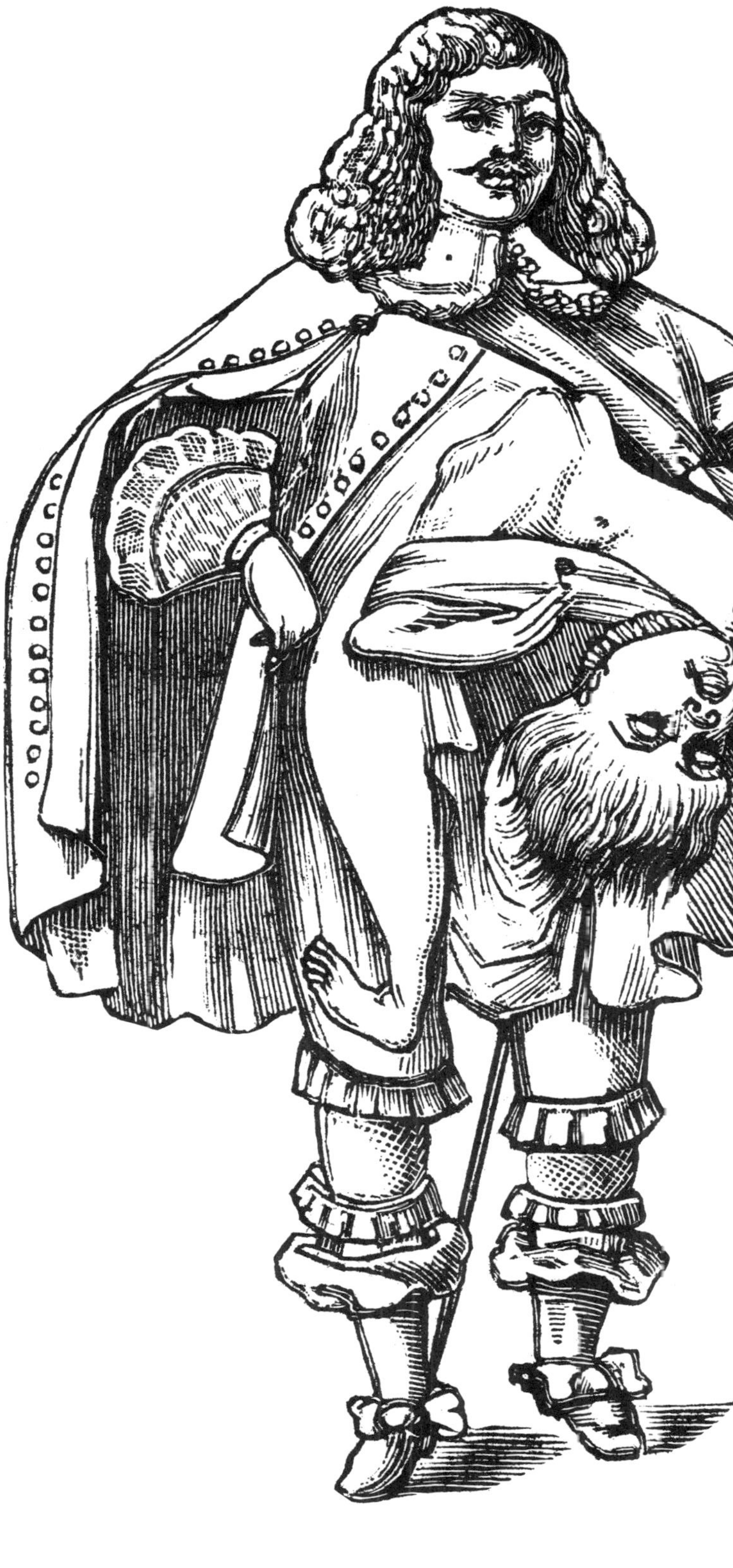

PHOCOMELIA

Phocomelia is a deformity in which hands and feet of usual size and habitually normal are supported by excessively short members which, in the majority of cases, seem to protrude directly from the body.

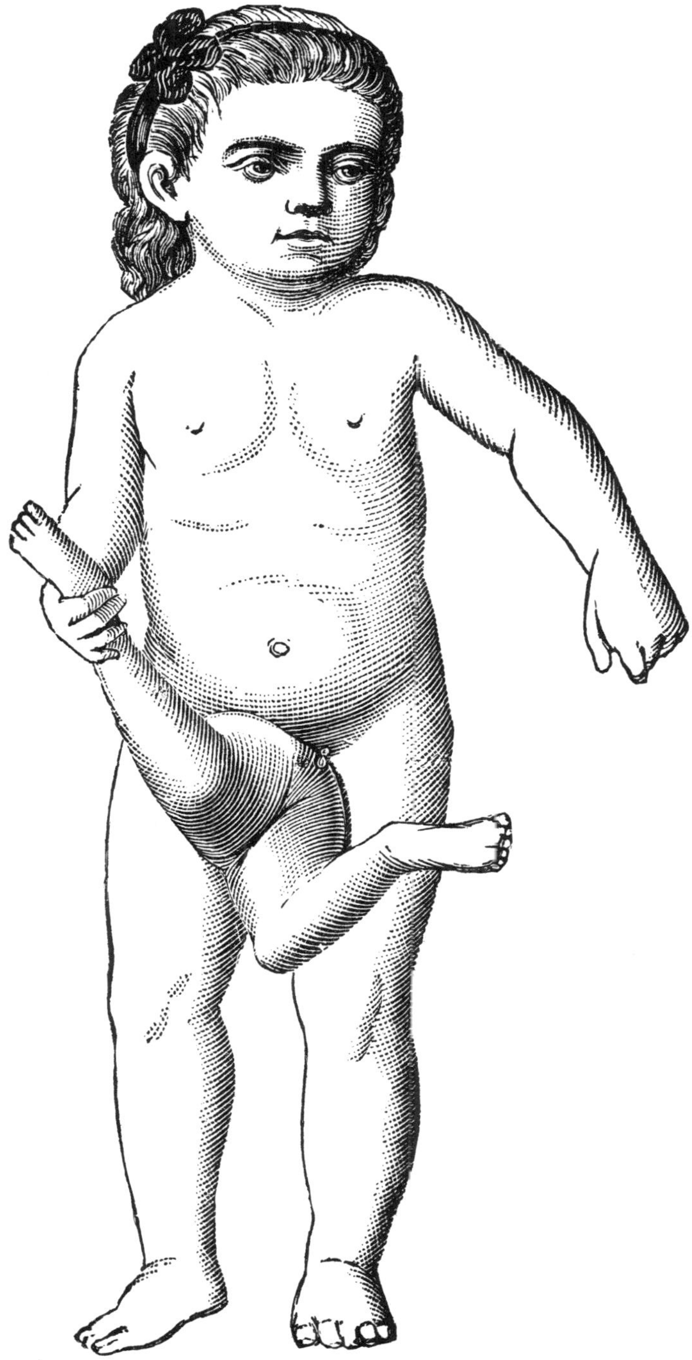

PELVIC PHOCOMELIA

This is a unique anomaly affecting all three segments of the limb. Single pelvic phocomelia seems more common than the deformity whereby both pelvic members are affected.

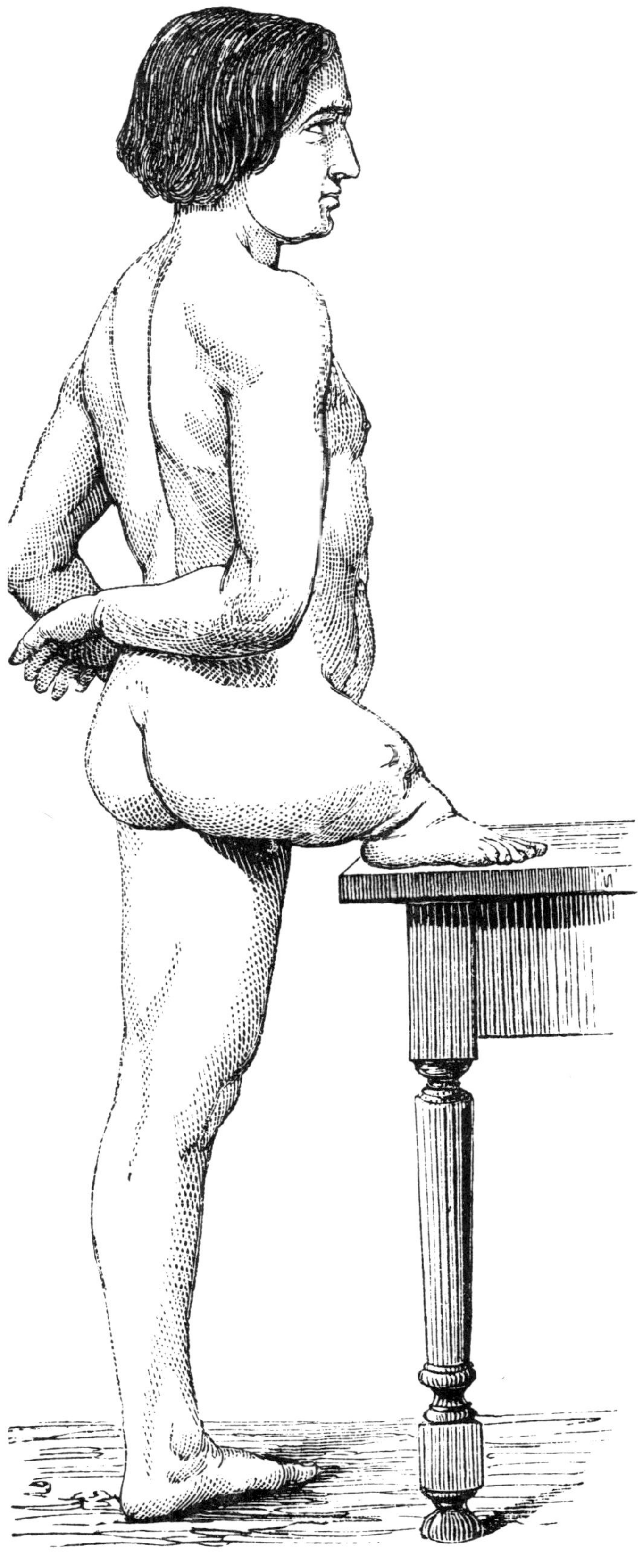

BI-ABDOMINAL ECTROMELIA AND ECTRODACTYLIA OF THE LEFT THORACIC LIMB

E. Dedout relates the fact that a young English lord born in this state became, thanks to the help of prostheses, one of the most intrepid fox-hunters in Ireland.

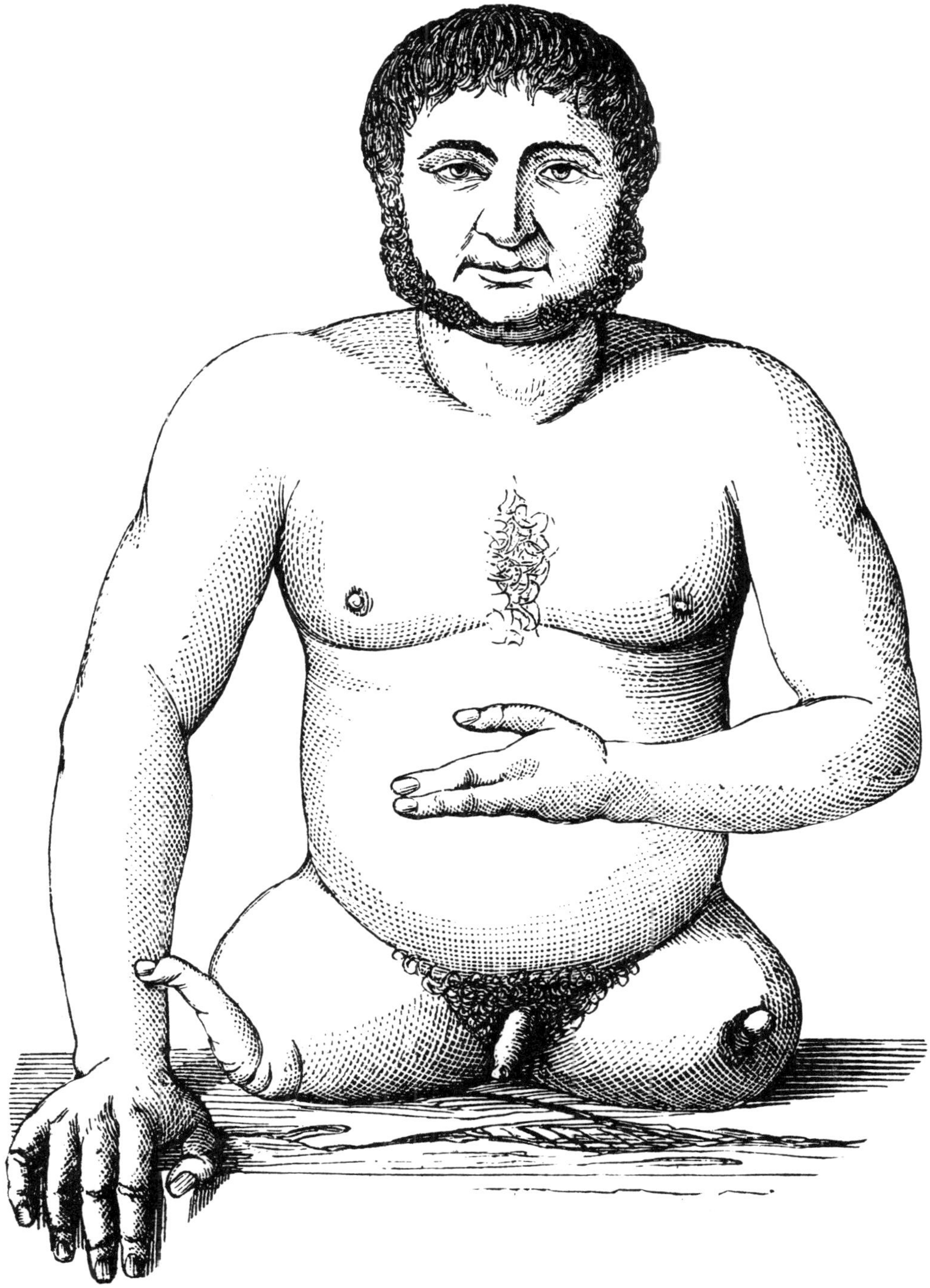

BITHORACIC HEMIMELIA AND UNILATERAL ABDOMINAL HEMINELIA

This subject has a rounded stump as upper right limb, a conical stump as upper left limb, and a rounded stump terminating the left thigh.

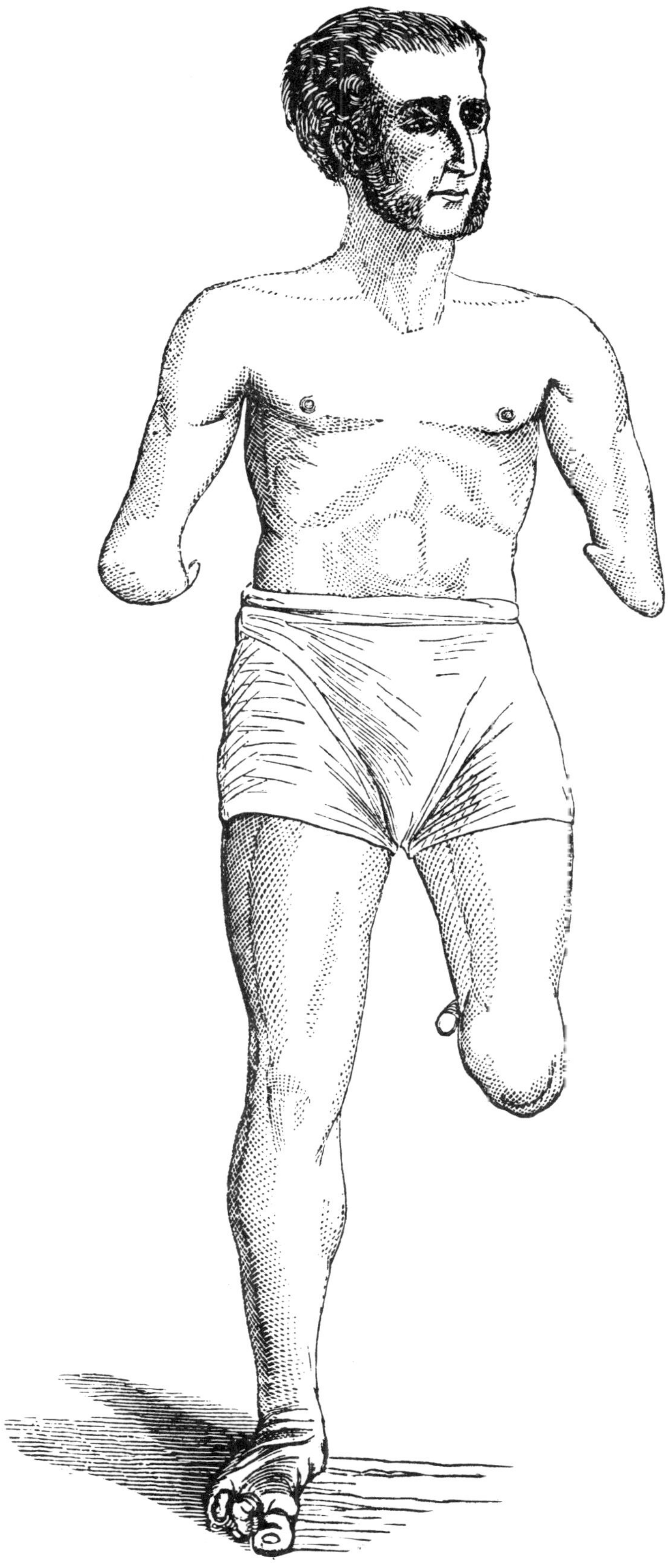

PYGOMELIA

Polymelian monsters are double monsters in which the parasite is reduced to one or a few limbs that insert themselves directly on the principal. In the case of the pygomelian type, the principal carries one or two supplementary limbs in the hypogastric region, inserted between the new limbs. Pygomelian monsters are not rare, at least not among birds.

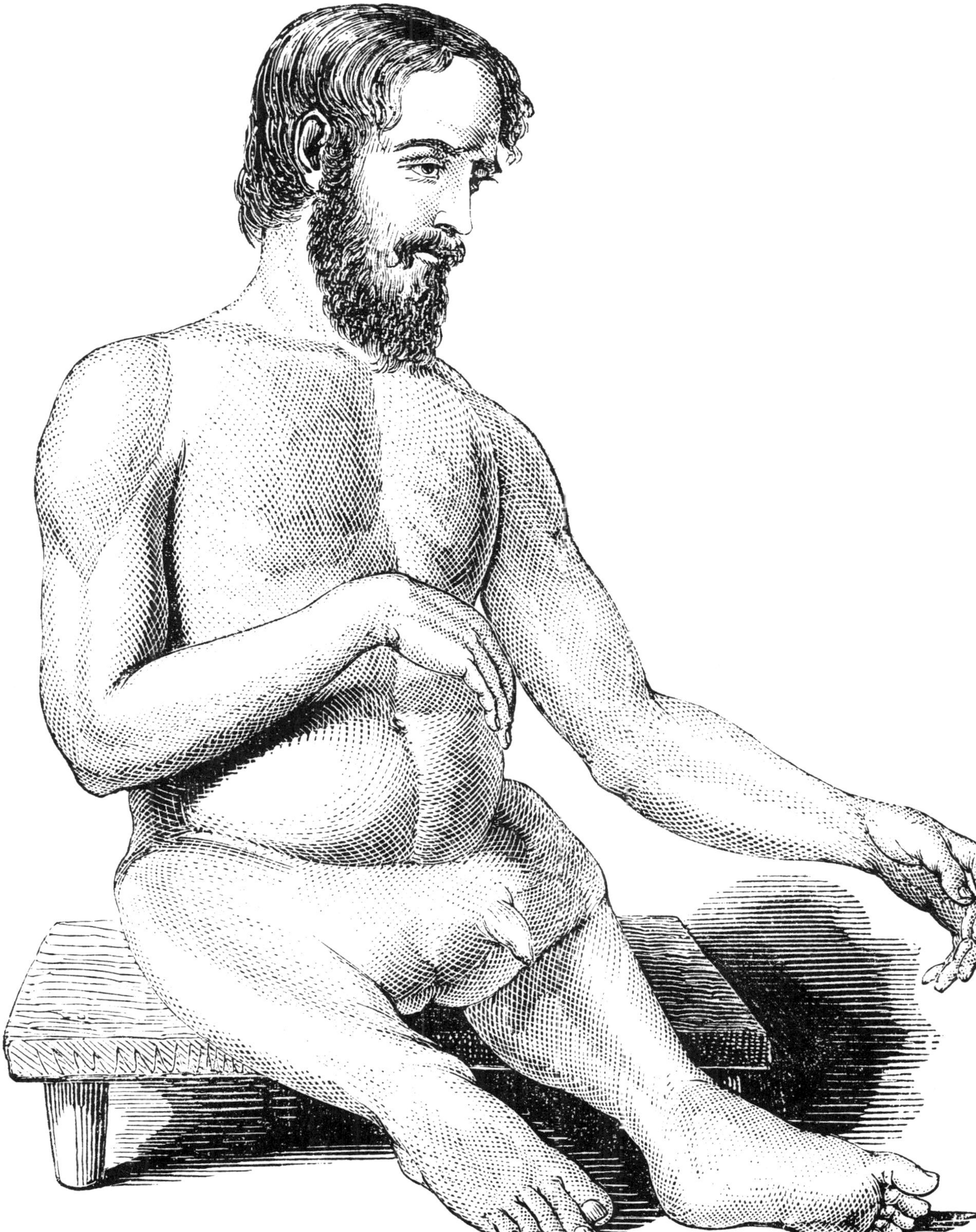

QUADRUPLE PHOCOMELIA

Considered from the point of view of their treatment, malformations resulting from the absence of bones, or of any other parts of the limbs, fall rather more within the competence of the manufacturer of artificial limbs, rather than within the surgeon's.

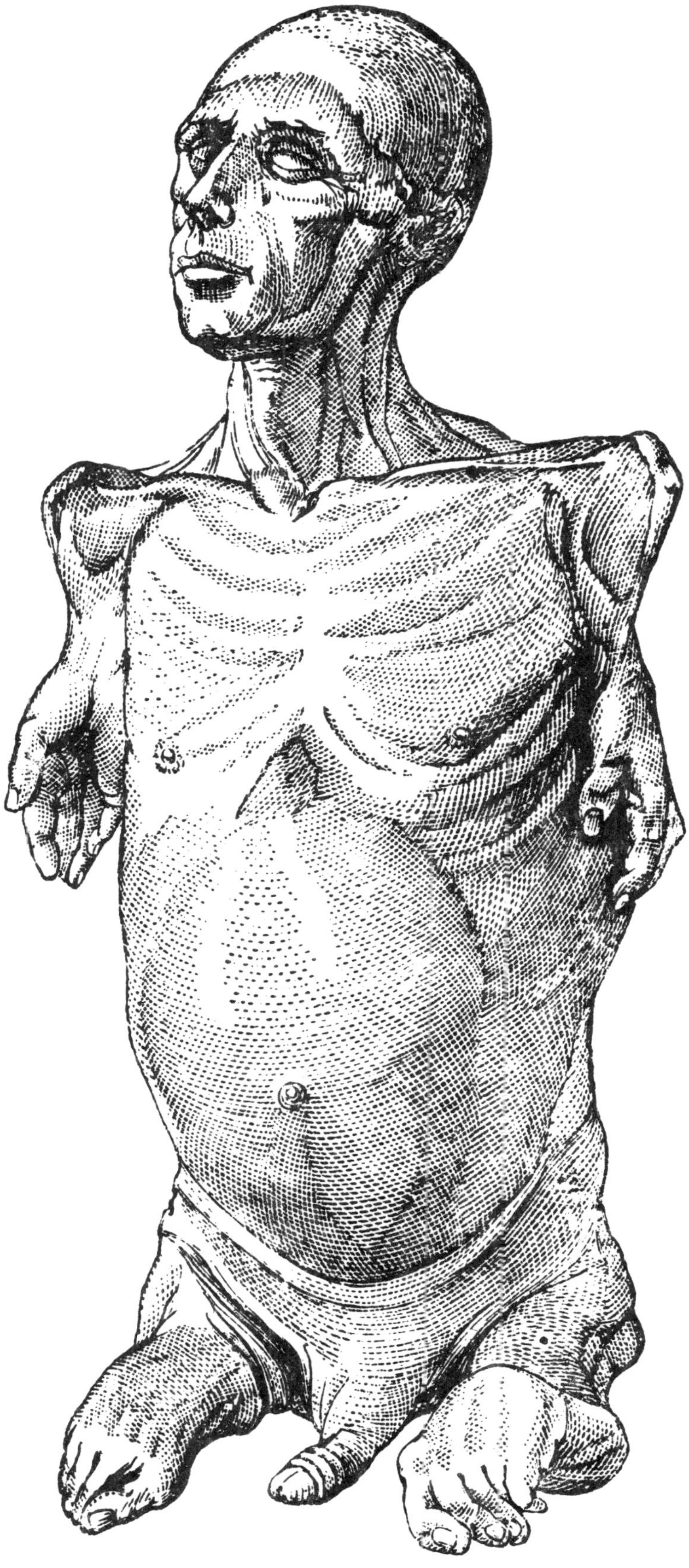

DOG MAN

Adrien Jeftichev, the Russian "dog man", is one of the most interesting cases of disorderly hair growth. Hypertrichosis is generally an hereditary ailment. The growth of the soft and woolly hair increases with age, and it is most pronounced on the face.

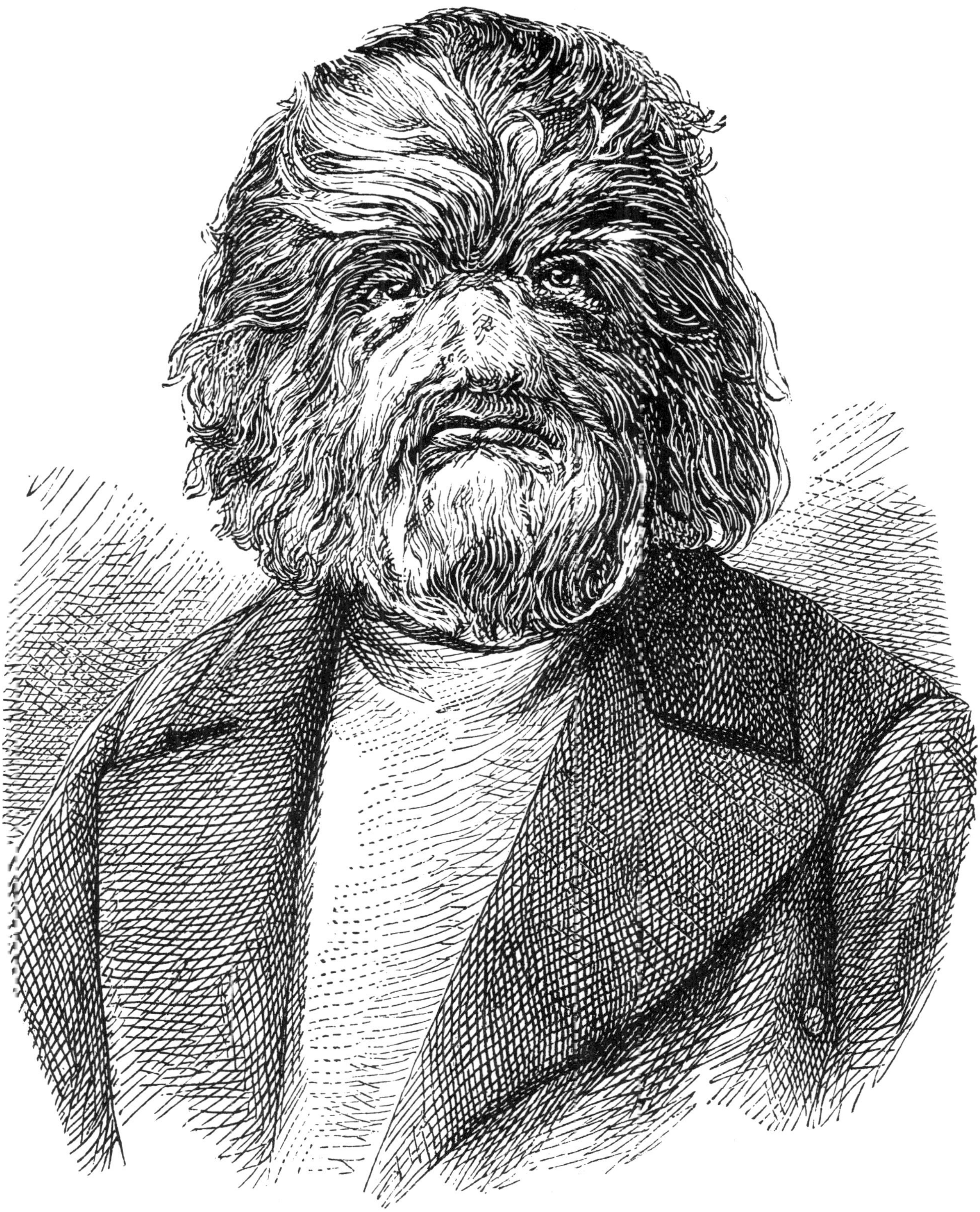

BEARDED LADY

On February 16, 1815, a person of dubious sex was presented to the society of the Faculty of Medicine in Paris. It was observed that Marie-Madeleine Lefort presented both masculine and feminine characteristics.

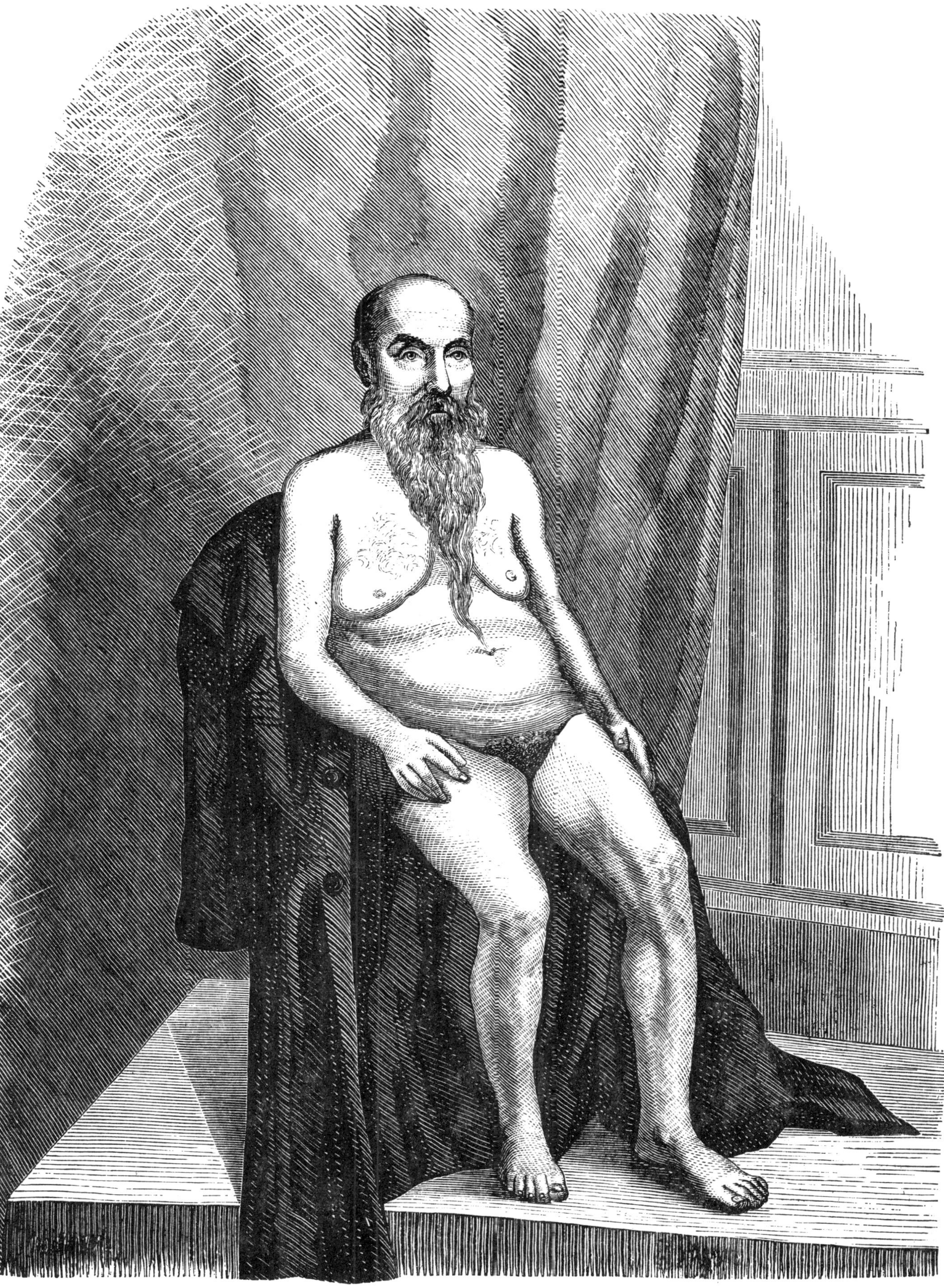

HERMAPHRODITE

This thirteen year old hermaphrodite is considered to belong to the feminine sex. There is no vagina, but the clitoris seems to be well developed and has an indentation and a prepuce above its vertex. Beneath, there is a hollow the size of a hazel-nut, leading to a small aperture from which the urine flows. The right testicle is very high and much smaller than the left one and, to feel it, one has to search carefully.

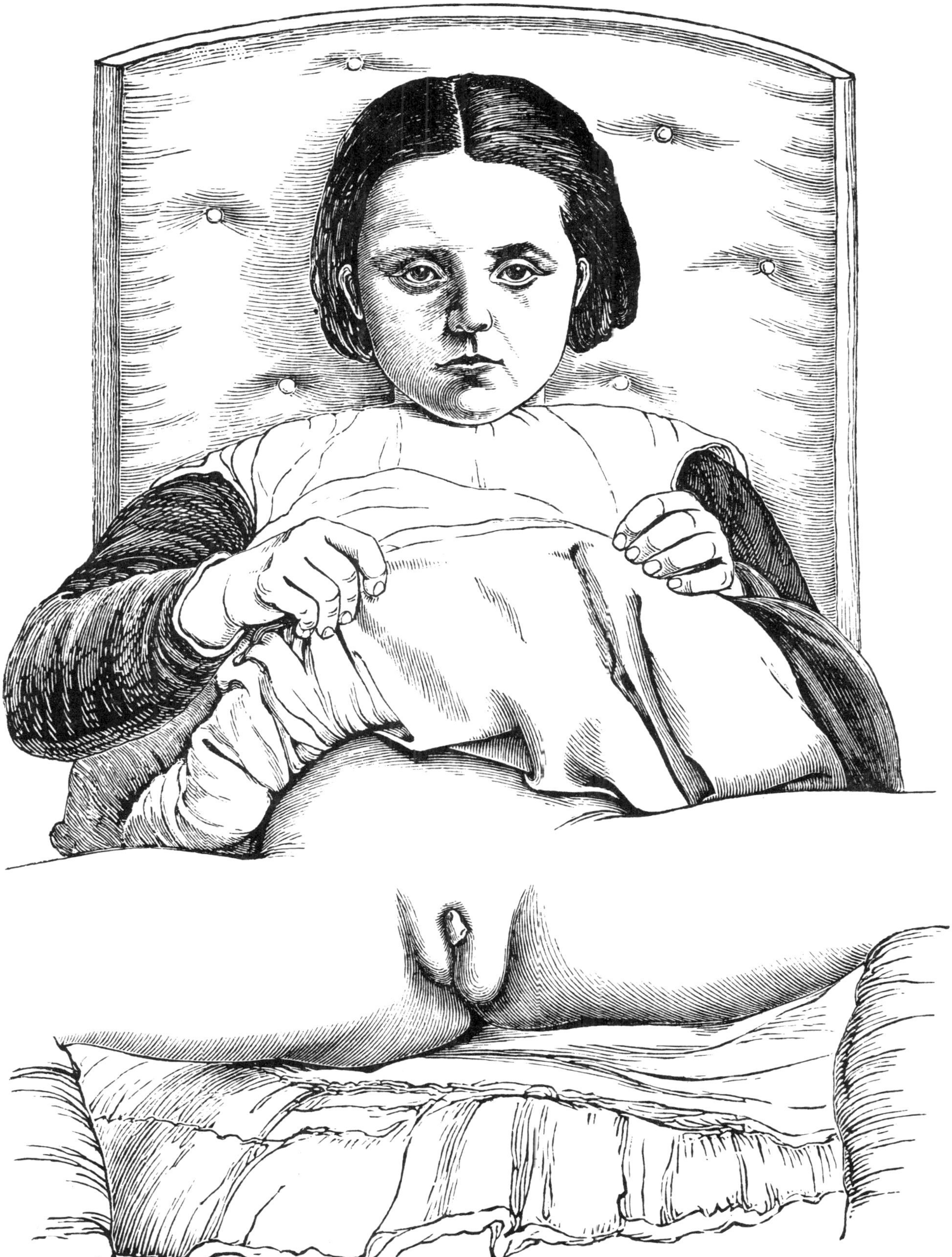